Contemporary Practice in Studio Art Therapy

Contemporary Practice in Studio Art Therapy discovers where studio practice stands in the profession today and reflects on how changing social, political, and economic contexts have influenced its ethos and development.

This is the first UK volume devoted to studio art therapy, and the writers explore what is meant by a studio approach and how they are adapting art-based practices in radical new ways and settings. It comprises three parts – *Part I: Frames of reference* explores how particular social, cultural, and political contexts have led to the discourses within practice; *Part II: Models of practice* gives accounts of current studio art therapy practice, describing rationale for working methods and providing a resource for practitioners; *Part III: Curating, exhibiting, and archiving* considers how the display and disposal of artworks, particularly relevant to studio approaches, may be thought about and implemented. The book includes chapters from North American authors who illustrate a trajectory of practice that has the potential to point to future developments.

The book will be essential reading for practitioners and students who are interested in taking a fresh perspective on art therapy and will be encouraged by new ways of thinking about the studio approach in today's changing world.

Christopher Brown is an artist and art therapist currently in private practice after retiring from careers in mental health and higher education.

Helen Omand is an artist and art therapist working in a therapeutic studio and as a lecturer at Goldsmiths, University of London.

This multi-authored book explores the history and development of studio-based art therapy in a diverse range of settings and from numerous theoretical perspectives. There is no comparable UK publication, and it makes a valuable and timely contribution to the literature. While its main readership is likely to be practicing arts therapists and students in training, this book contains much that will also be of interest to artists, mental health workers, and practitioners from related disciplines.

David Edwards, *artist, retired HCPC registered art therapist, and author of the book Art Therapy*

Contemporary Practice in Studio Art Therapy offers fresh, compelling, multifaceted perspectives on the physical and conceptual significance of the studio in art therapy. Readers are challenged to consider how historical, social, and political contexts continue to shape such practices.

Catherine Hyland Moon, *Professor, School of the Art Institute of Chicago*

This vital and timely book places the studio at the heart of art therapy, updating the studio's historic significance with descriptions of innovative new practices, much of which arises to meet the needs of people suffering the adverse effects of socio-economic and political realities. The thoughtful and wide-ranging chapters impress on the reader the centrality of art and art making and the significance of art therapy studios as inclusive, adaptable, and creative places.

Dean Reddick, *art therapist with Latimer Community Art Therapy; co-editor of, Art Therapy in the Early Years: Therapeutic Interventions with Infants, Toddlers and their Families*

Art therapy practice initially developed in studios, and this book is an inspiring reminder of their contemporary relevance. The clear structure, engaging chapters, and breadth of contexts and client groups make it an essential read. This book will inspire many to explore studio art therapy practice.

Val Huet, *PhD, Director of Research, British Association of Art Therapists, and trustee of the Adamson Collection Trust*

Given the importance of different styles of studio to the development and practice of therapeutic art, it is perhaps surprising that there are not more books exploring this important subject. This book will help to fill this notable gap.

Susan Hogan, *Professor of Arts and Health, University of Derby*

This book offers a truly thought-provoking view of 'studio art therapy'. Including much-needed contributions from both UK and US practitioners, it presents a complex portrait of changing times, practices, values, and ways of thinking about an eternally evolving field, and the spaces where people can create and become themselves.

Judith A. Rubin, *PhD, President of Expressive Media, author of six books, and Director of thirteen films about art therapy*

Contemporary Practice in Studio Art Therapy

Edited by Christopher Brown and Helen Omand

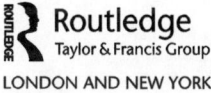

Routledge
Taylor & Francis Group

LONDON AND NEW YORK

First published 2022
by Routledge
2 Park Square, Milton Park, Abingdon, Oxon OX14 4RN

and by Routledge
605 Third Avenue, New York, NY 10158

Routledge is an imprint of the Taylor & Francis Group, an informa business

British Library Cataloguing-in-Publication Data
A catalogue record for this book is available from the British Library

Library of Congress Cataloging-in-Publication Data
Names: Brown, Christopher, editor. | Omand, Helen, editor.
Title: Contemporary practice in studio art therapy / edited by Christopher Brown and Helen Omand.
Description: Milton Park, Abingdon, Oxon ; New York, NY : Routledge, 2022. | Includes bibliographical references and index.
Identifiers: LCCN 2021040371 (print) | LCCN 2021040372 (ebook) | ISBN 9780367558932 (hardback) | ISBN 9780367558925 (paperback) | ISBN 9781003095606 (ebook)
Subjects: LCSH: Art therapy. | Art therapists—Training of.
Classification: LCC RC489.A7 C68 2022 (print) | LCC RC489.A7 (ebook) | DDC 616.89/1656—dc23/eng/20211012
LC record available at https://lccn.loc.gov/2021040371
LC ebook record available at https://lccn.loc.gov/2021040372

ISBN: 978-0-367-55893-2 (hbk)
ISBN: 978-0-367-55892-5 (pbk)
ISBN: 978-1-003-09560-6 (ebk)

DOI: 10.4324/9781003095606

Typeset in Times New Roman
by Apex CoVantage, LLC

Contents

Notes on contributors

Mary Andrus is an assistant professor and programme director of the Art Therapy Program in the Graduate School of Education and Counselling at Lewis and Clark in Portland, Oregon. Her scholarship focus is on expanding clinical practice beyond traditional practices, the use of film in reintegration, and the implications of art therapy in the treatment of individual and collective trauma.

Zoë Armstrong is co-owner of a counselling service in Yukon Territory, Canada. She is an exhibiting artist and art therapist with a focus on trauma, grief and loss, and crisis intervention. Gifted with profound dyslexia and ADD, she has a special interest in neurodiversity and gender and uses the pronouns she/her/hers.

Christopher Brown is retired from careers as an art therapist working in NHS adult mental health and teaching on art therapy trainings. He now works in private practice and continues to make and exhibit art. He is a founding member of the open access journal *ATOL: Art Therapy OnLine*.

Philippa Brown was Professional Lead of Art Therapy at the School of Creative Arts, University of Hertfordshire, from 1994 to 2016. She now works as an art therapy supervisor and a Health and Care Professions Council Visitor. She is also a visiting lecturer at various higher education institutions.

Dalaila Bumanglag formed an interest in studio approaches through her involvement with Studio Upstairs as a trainee and volunteer art therapist. She completed her research dissertation on the therapeutic value of the open studio approach. Her interests include working in special educational needs and cancer care.

Kristen Catchpole is an art psychotherapist who has specialised in working with families presenting with complex needs in court-ordered residential assessment. She has managed therapy teams inside primary education and worked with vulnerable adults with sustained brain injuries. She is a lecturer at Goldsmiths, University of London, and also employed by a charity working in paediatric care in the NHS.

Annamaria Cavaliero is an art psychotherapist working in the field of adult mental health. A graduate from Goldsmiths, University of London, she subsequently worked there as a part-time lecturer on the MA Art Psychotherapy course. She is also a practising artist.

Tessa Dalley is an experienced art therapist and child and adolescent psychotherapist currently working in independent practice with children, young people, and families. She has worked in a variety of settings and published widely on art therapy and child psychotherapy. She is a clinical supervisor to other practising therapists and Chair of the Squiggle Foundation, dedicated to the work of Donald Winnicott.

David Fried is an artist and art therapist. Born in 1958, he grew up in Copenhagen and London and trained at Hornsey College of Art, The Royal College of Art, and St Albans School of Art. He has worked in NHS Adult Mental Health and in the independent sector. He has spent his life working with art both for itself and as a therapeutic endeavour.

Douglas Gill was a performance artist, community artist, and art therapist before training in psychoanalytic psychotherapy. His interests in the arts and psychoanalysis continue on from transforming the arts into a psychoanalytic frame to exploring the rich dialogue they have with contemporary culture. He lives in London, where he is in private practice.

Lynn Kapitan is a professor and founding director of art therapy at Mount Mary University in Milwaukee, WI (USA). A past president of the American Art Therapy Association and former editor of their journal *Art Therapy*, she has written extensively on art therapy, often drawing from her cross-cultural research experience and work in diverse settings.

Bobby Lloyd is an artist, HCPC registered art therapist, supervisor, lecturer, and CEO of Art Refuge, with a background in NHS and community settings, UK and internationally. Through Art Refuge she is increasingly interested in the roles of art and art therapy in relation to displacement, community, crisis support, and social justice.

Claire Manson has worked as an art psychotherapist for over forty years in both the NHS and the independent sector; including pro bono work in human rights organisations – the Medical Foundation for the Care of Victims of Torture, Baobab Centre for Young Survivors in Exile, and the Cotton Tree Trust.

Jon Martyn trained as an art psychotherapist at Goldsmiths, University of London. He has worked in Freedom from Torture's open art studio, for Leicester's personality disorder service, at the London Art Therapy Centre, and as a lecturer at Goldsmiths. Along with Tania Kaczynski, he co-founded the New Art Studio for refugees and asylum seekers in 2014.

Patsy McMahon attended Hornsey College of Art at eighteen years of age in the 1960s and Chelsea College of Art in her forties, after having a family. In her art practice she is interested in the techniques ordinary people developed to use with imagination to work against tyranny. She is interested in the space between things.

Helen Omand is an art therapist who works in a therapeutic art studio and teaches on the MA Art Psychotherapy at Goldsmiths, University of London. She is interested in the relationship between personal art practice and working as an art therapist, and she exhibits with a collective of artists and art therapists.

Kristina Page has degrees in fine art and art psychotherapy as well as a diploma in group work from the Institute of Group Analysis. She is a clinical supervisor at the Ben Uri Gallery and Museum, a studio manager at Studio Upstairs, and also works in private practice.

Steve Pratt is an artist and art psychotherapist working in the forensic setting and in private practice.

Simon Richardson has been working in a range of health and social care settings since 1996. He currently works as a housing progression coordinator for a homeless charity in London and volunteers with a community arts in health project. Simon maintains his own art practice and regularly participates in group exhibitions.

Miriam Usiskin is an HCPC registered art therapist, supervisor, and senior lecturer, MA Art Therapy, University of Hertfordshire. With a background in NHS acute settings, she now specialises in displacement, crisis support, and resilience. A lead member of the Art Refuge team since 2016, she is currently pursuing an educational doctorate on its work.

Ben Wakeling is an artist and founder of the Outsider Gallery and the Art School of Hackney Wick Life Drawing in London. He is a guest arts lecturer at the University of the West of England, Bristol. He has worked with the North London Forensic Service for Barnet Enfield and Haringey Mental Health Trust.

Chris Wood works as an art therapist in the NHS and is an HE trainer and researcher in Sheffield, though no longer a course leader. She is inspired by the life stories of service users, students, and people working in mental health services. Her publications are listed on the ORCID system.

Foreword

In a modern world saturated with flashing lights, advertising slogans with imagery that is often manufactured or digitally manipulated, alongside social media becoming one of the main forms of communication, it is a pleasure that we have this book that takes time to look, to reflect, to contemplate the permanence and lasting importance of an image and the studio space in which it is created. The internal world of the artist comes alive in the private process of making and doing which gives symbolic form to an experience that can then be shared. In a move away from psychoanalytic ideas, the authors invite us to consider the therapeutic value of this experience by revisiting the healing power of art as a foundation of art therapy practice.

The profound influence of formative writers such as Berger (1972) and Fuller (1981a, 1981b) challenged attitudes to art appreciation in new 'ways of seeing' and understanding aesthetic response. In a foreword to one of the early books on art therapy, Fuller (1984) points to the shift in understanding when psychoanalysts, such as Marion Milner, confronted the fact that art is necessary for the development of creativity and health. He also commented on the way in which advanced technological societies tend to marginalise the production of art and 'to seal over this third area' which Winnicott described as the 'location of human experience'. At the same time, Edward Adamson, who many regard as the founder of art therapy, was working in an art studio with traumatised soldiers. His containing, thoughtful approach to the contemplation of the art image, when meaning and understanding grows in the presence of another, is well documented in this book. Using the studio as a therapeutic and physical space 'where people have the liberty to think and speak: aesthetically, emotionally, socially, and to remain silent if they wish' (Chapter 5) subsequently became the bedrock of art therapy philosophy and practice. The studio remains safe and the same – an evolving, creative, emerging place with emphasis on being 'art focussed' as a 'lived experience'. As thought is framed and contained in this way, the studio space can exist as a mental space in the mind of the self as well as the other.

This visionary book describes how a studio can embrace marginalised communities and people who may be homeless, alienated by social and political conflict, displaced, or in a confused state of psychic unreality. Art making maintains and develops relationships between individuals and communities to share understanding, promote social action and change. Innovation has tensions, and by tracing the ideas of the studio model through the passage of time, the different contributors, currently working in a variety of settings, give a strong voice to contemporary practice and moving forward in the future. As well as stability, the concept of studio is both portable and permanent, and, by working in more transient and fragile environments, the traditional studio model will adapt to the demands of these changing landscapes. However marginal, as the final part on curating, exhibiting, and archiving demonstrates, art reaches across borders, cultures, and language and will continue to speak to the many deeply personal stories of human experience which do not disappear like words.

Tessa Dalley

References

Berger, J. (1972) *Ways of Seeing*. London. Penguin Books.

Fuller, P. (1981a) *Art and Psychoanalysis*. London. Writers and Readers.

Fuller, P. (1981b) *Seeing Berger: A Re-Evaluation of Ways of Seeing*. London. Writers and Readers.

Fuller, P. (1984) Foreword in Dalley, T. (ed) *Art as Therapy. An Introduction to the Use of Art as a Therapeutic Technique*. London. Routledge.

Acknowledgements

First and foremost, we thank our contributing authors, for their time and dedication in producing such rich chapters and for working with us as editors.

Huge thanks to Andrea Gilroy, who not only championed the project but also provided critical thinking on our ideas and gave detailed comments on Chapter 1. Special thanks go to the following art therapists who so generously took the time to respond to our questions regarding the possibility of a 'psychoanalytic turn' within the profession: Caroline Case, Jane Dudley, Katherine Killick, Jacky Mahony, Joy Schaverien, Robin Tipple, Diane Waller. Their contributions, which were more extensive than we have used, helped us develop our thinking about wider issues within the book. Thanks to the following for their comments and insights on reading draft chapters: Sarah Bakewell, Dean Reddick, and Diana Velada. We also thank Lynn Kapitan for her assistance and knowledge of North American practice. Special thanks to Chris Allen for his sterling work in preparing the images. Last but not least, we thank Joanne Forshaw at Routledge for her support throughout the process of bringing the book into being.

Introduction

Christopher Brown and Helen Omand

This book is the first UK volume devoted to studio art therapy. It explores the contexts in which studio practice developed, its various approaches, and its current use in a variety of settings – some of which operate in the margins of art therapy practice and bring new ways of thinking about the studio approach.

We wanted to produce this book for several reasons. First, having worked in studio settings, we were curious about what had been written on the subject in the UK (see Omand and Bumanglag, Chapter 2), and we wanted to hear from other art therapists about their practice. We wondered to what extent our experience of the value of studio space, with an emphasis on ongoing art making processes, was shared by others. Second, we were curious to know if studio approaches were more commonplace than current literature would suggest. It has been our experience as practitioners, supervisors, and educators that it is not unusual for art therapists and trainees to be asked to run 'studio' groups or groups based on an 'open studio' model. We felt, perhaps like other art therapists, that we had an implicit understanding of what was meant by these terms, but we wondered what assumptions we held and how they might be usefully unpicked. For example, what is meant by a studio approach and how are studio groups different from other art therapy groups and practices? Where is studio art therapy practice located today – who is doing it and why? A not uncommon question is, where is the 'therapy' happening in studio art therapy – is it even 'proper' art therapy at all? We wondered if there had been some kind of gap in the shared knowledge of the profession; a 'looking away' from studio models of working, we were curious about why this had happened in the UK and less so in other countries.

This book highlights why ideas from studio art therapy are particularly relevant in the current art therapy climate where there is renewed interest in turning back to the art in art therapy. To understand why this is happening, and where studio approaches fit within this, our contributors explore the contextual changes that have brought about new ways of working. Indeed, much of the innovative work described in the book has arisen in response to human suffering brought about by changing social, political, and economic situations. The chapters trace the evolution of this development and discover where studio practice is located today.

DOI: 10.4324/9781003095606-1

The studio

Why *studio* art therapy? you ask. In our attempt to answer this question, we need to consider what a studio is, why it is important for artists, and what implications this may have for the practice of art therapy. We start with a statement from art historian John Milner that addresses the first of these:

> The studio is no more than a container, a kind of equipment, a room in which to paint or sculpt, a necessary space. In its isolation the artist watches a painting or sculpture, adjusts it, instinctively responsive to pigments, colours and materials, resolving their conflicts, bringing them together. In this way the studio is also an arena in which controlled yet instinctive and unpremeditated discovery unfolds. It is both a space apart and an essential arena for action.
>
> (Milner, 2009: 65)

This example suggests a rather privileged space, based on European and North American ideas of what 'art' is, something outside of everyday life, as opposed to art being embedded in communal craft activities, architecture, or religious practices for example. Clearly, the history of fine art has shaped a particular idea of the quintessential artist's studio. Moon has pointed out that in art therapy this sort of studio space is more myth than reality, and that an art therapy studio is more likely to be 'a studio smacked down, dead center, in the middle of life' (2002: 68). Certainly, the communal aspects of many art therapy studios mean that rather than being sealed off from life they are meeting points – between the group, the therapist, and the wider social context as well as between the individual and their own art making. But Milner's idea of a space apart is more than just the physical space, which nowadays may be as diverse as a laptop, a library, a converted office building, depending on the means of production being employed, within communities or public spaces (Harrison, 2009). The non-physical aspects are just as important; it offers a space for reflection, for imagination, for the internal world to find external form, a point not lost on the title chosen for the original journal of the British Association of Art Therapists – *Inscape*. An art therapy studio may also hold the idea of a refuge from distress or an oasis of calm, which may be true or may be an idealisation that denies the disturbance and tumult to be found within it (see Wood, Chapter 3; Kapitan, Chapter 4; Cavaliero, Chapter 13).

So, the space in which art therapy takes place is important and part of the setting for art therapy (see Brown, Chapter 7). For the early UK pioneers this was most often a studio equipped for making art within an asylum or a therapeutic community. As the profession developed, towards the end of the twentieth century, changing healthcare contexts meant many studios closed or moved into community settings. The expense of real estate became a consideration for institutions such as the NHS; however, the idea of multi-use rooms was driven not only economically but also ideologically as part of egalitarian thinking around multidisciplinary working in teams. Once the setting becomes compromised there is potential for erosion of other boundaries and loss of containment for the work (see

Killick's comments in Chapter 2; Brown, Chapter 7). Some of our contributors explore ways in which a studio ethos is particularly useful in less-than-ideal settings (see Lloyd and Usiskin, Chapter 8; Wakeling, Chapter 10; Pratt, Chapter 11).

The frame

The development of studio art therapy privileged ideas from art education and social justice, which led to the construction of a frame that differs markedly from psychodynamic orthodoxy. The professionalisation of art therapy has taken it on a journey through differing social and political contexts to where it is currently located. This location has become like a market, where art therapy can be seen to align itself to a variety of competing ideologies, each influencing practice, all hoping to attract custom; for example, psychoanalysis, psychology, cognitive behavioural therapy, mentalisation, mindfulness, etc. The issue of defining the frame for studio art therapy is a pressing one for art therapists in the current climate, where a range of disciplines may be competing for an institution's funding across a whole spectrum of therapies and arts in health initiatives. We need to be able to say what it is, how it works, and what makes it a useful intervention.

Some of the elements that make up a studio ethos are a focus on sustained art making over time rather than producing art for interpretation, interactions often concerned more with processes and materials than eliciting meaning, nonintrusive engagement or ways of relating that promote an individual's agency to choose how to engage and at what pace, the open nature of the space – all contribute to an ethos that place the art and the person in a more human context as opposed to a clinical one (see Omand and Bumanglag, Chapter 2). Crucially, these elements have also influenced what are generally known as 'open studio groups' or 'studio based open groups', which are commonplace in UK art therapy today, being held on wards in institutions or as part of outpatient or community services. We trace the origins of these elements in the work of early pioneers in art therapy and consider how the practice of art therapy was influenced by the antipsychiatry movement, analytical psychology, and psychoanalysis amongst others (see Brown and Omand, Chapter 1; Omand and Bumanglag, Chapter 2). Does history show a move away from art-based studio practice and a turn towards a more psychotherapeutic practice? Did the profession abandon its artistic and libertarian roots in the process? And is there now a resurgence of interest in studio art therapy or did it never go away? These are questions we hope to answer and draw conclusions from that are relevant to the emerging contexts of contemporary practice.

A further aspect of the frame of studio art therapy is that work made within this frame is sometimes publicly exhibited and so taken beyond the perimeter of the frame into a public context. The ethics and considerations behind the display and exhibiting of artworks have been largely neglected, despite their importance across diverse art therapy practices. We hope to redress this by devoting a section of the book to exploring the issues that arise when the art is taken out of the frame (see Armstrong, Chapter 9; Page, Chapter 15; Martyn, Chapter 16; Andrus, Chapter 17; Brown and Omand, Chapter 19).

The social context

The art therapy studio and the ideas that underpin it provide a context within which ethical issues around 'mental health' may be highlighted and worked with, such as problems around the pathologising of behaviours and psychiatric diagnosis, the location and meaning of 'madness' or 'normality' in society, and the nature of human distress. A growing body of literature points out that art therapists are not exempt from working within medical diagnostic paradigms; this may take the form of an expectation that a person with knowledge 'reads' a picture according to aesthetic qualities of the work and its symbolic content, then relates this back to a person's individual psychopathology (Tipple, 2003; Hogan, 2016; Talwar, 2019). The long tradition of egalitarianism and a less interpretative stance in studio art therapy can contribute to ideas about where the meaning of a person's art resides, to shift power imbalances in the hierarchical divide between clinician as knowledge holder and the service user's lived experience; for example, a focus on the personal meaning of an artwork for the artist rather than a psychodynamic interpretation from the therapist. Other literature, particularly from the US, has emphasised art therapy studios as social spaces for empowerment (Moon, 2016; see also Kapitan, Chapter 4). A focus on the wider social and political context impacting on a person rather than locating problems within the individual also redresses clinical and social imbalances of power (see Armstrong, Chapter 9; Andrus, Chapter 17). Hogan has pointed out that art therapy has roots in the tradition of moral treatment of mental illness that emerged from Utilitarian philosophy in the nineteenth century (2001). Twentieth-century ideas of social justice, influenced by the antipsychiatry movement and the Frankfurt school, for example, link studio art therapy directly to current ethical debates in art therapy about power and clinician–service user hierarchies (see Brown and Omand, Chapter 1; Manson, Gill and Fried, Chapter 5; Armstrong, Chapter 9; Omand and McMahon, Chapter 12).

Studio groups today often work with people who have been marginalised by society, such as those whose experience of mainstream services has made them wary of further engagement, or who are at a time of crisis, or who have been displaced and are in urgent need of intervention. People in these situations may be unlikely to engage with conventional therapeutic services or not have the verbal or symbolic resources needed for expressing themselves in other settings. Many of the chapter authors address these controversial topics (see Lloyd and Usiskin, Chapter 8; Armstrong, Chapter 9; Wakeling, Chapter 10; Pratt, Chapter 11; Martyn, Chapter 16).

The impact of neoliberal policies of austerity on the economies of caring professions, perhaps a swing away from emphasis on psychoanalytic ideas and a turning back to the healing power of art in art therapy, pressures to align with scientific models of evidence, a growing need for approaches that can meet current market expectations – are all topics explored by our contributors. We have two chapter authors from the United States and one from Canada, where the context in which art therapy developed differs from that in Britain. Their contributions provide a counterpoint to UK practice and offer ideas on future directions this practice might take, emphasising socially and ethically informed studio practices with a focus on empowerment and social justice.

The virtual studio

We have been editing this book during the global pandemic of COVID-19. This has given us opportunity to consider the loss of a physical space in which to meet our clients and how online working may impact on practice, both positively and negatively. Perhaps the hardest aspect of therapy to replicate virtually is intimacy and much of the embodied experience from encounters in person is absent on videoconferencing platforms such as Zoom. This may, however, be welcomed by those who prefer a cooler, more distant connection. Another shift is in the power dynamic when the therapist is in the client's room not the other way round, which may feel intrusive for the client and indeed for the therapist if having to work from home rather than an office. The freedom of open group boundaries is harder to replicate on Zoom, where instead of moving where we please around a room, speech is directed to the whole group and only one conversation can happen at a time. This and other concerns about looking and being seen may make Zoom prohibitively uncomfortable for some (see Omand, 2023).

How to see the art properly is another concern for studio approaches online. The visceral qualities of an ongoing art making process are harder to witness online, and the way artworks resonate in a group is harder to appreciate. Clients may not have access to a desktop computer and be using a smartphone, where people and images are reduced to small windows, and here access to resources and space can also bring up inequalities that affect the online experience.

Concluding remarks

Whatever the future may hold in terms of space and place for art therapy, we believe the ethos presented in this book will play a part. We hope the chapters that follow stimulate thinking and debate about the setting for art therapy in the forthcoming fifth phase of our history (see Wood, Chapter 3). The chapters in this book locate studio art therapy firmly in the present as a set of practices that are art-based, accessible, and bring people together in therapeutic studio spaces that are often improvised, from the communal dining area of a homeless shelter to a table in a refugee encampment, a hospital ward, or a graffiti wall. Not all authors have the advantages of a permanent space, and a theme of the book is how studio approaches lend themselves to application in radical new ways and communal situations.

Authors report outcomes that vary from expression, containment, processing of emotions, relating to others, development of a sense of self, agency, empowerment, and social justice, and in this last, the US seems to be leading the way. We see, in line with the history of the profession, that the author's theoretical outlook will subtly affect the way studio art therapy is conceived of. For example, Richardson cites Gel's work on art as agency for an art-based coming into being (Chapter 18); Page's group analytic thinking is applied to curating a wall of images in the studio (Chapter 15); Omand and McMahon negotiate the language they use when considering their artworks in the intersubjective space (Chapter 12); Armstrong employs a socially informed community empowerment approach (Chapter 9). These authors draw on theory that helps understand the art and the studio space in ways other than art in service of psychodynamic interpretation of the client's inner world. That said, the chapters in the book are mostly not theory heavy, and practice is notably focused around interest in how art is used, often innovatively. For example, the inmate of the segregation unit who pushed drawings under the door (Pratt, Chapter 11), a group painting as a starting process for young offenders (Wakeling, Chapter 10), a mother and baby playing with art materials (Catchpole, Chapter 14), or in the evocative tapping of old-fashioned typewriters used by refugees and migrants (Lloyd and Usiskin, Chapter 8).

This is in keeping with the artistic roots of studio art therapy. In the UK, a long history of studio practice by artists in psychiatric settings aligns it with libertarian attitudes of freedom, where patients are human beings and styles of relating can be straightforward and everyday rather than jargonistic. In the US, the history of studios is found in radical community arts, where studio art therapy has a more established ethos of democracy, collectivity, and accessibility, and the therapist identity may be more artist than 'clinician' and the 'patient' is relocated to artist (Moon, 2016). These approaches emphasise a health rather than illness model and thus take a political stance (see Brown and Omand, Chapter 1; Omand and Bumanglag, Chapter 2). Some authors notice the possibility of a more levelled power dynamic between the 'client' and the art therapist in the studio. They draw attention to the thinking around this and issues of hierarchy and power in therapeutic encounters. A history of oppressive practices in psychiatry, and of course in a wider sense politically and socially, has meant these are pressing ethical issues for art therapists working in institutions or in community settings. We were struck by the willingness of some authors to acknowledge their own lived experience, for example, how the therapist's trauma meets the patient's (Pratt, Chapter 11). We were also struck by the strong presence of the 'client voice' in others, from interview transcripts (Catchpole, Chapter 14; Martyn, Chapter 16) to a co-authored chapter (Omand and McMahon, Chapter 12).

One of the things that emerges from this book is the adaptable nature of the open studio group in the UK, where it exists in institutions such as psychiatric hospitals and young offender institutes, in community settings where populations and membership shifts, and as a response to crisis. It places the agency with the person, who can choose when and how much to engage in the group at their own pace. A studio is a way of being together on your own terms, making or not making art, talking or not talking. An art-based approach can reach across to those who might not engage in conventional therapy. A space to make art may seem deceptively simple but can involve the therapist negotiating complex institutional dynamics; spaces just to 'be' and to 'be' together, to feel and think and create are rare and may be resisted by a defensive institution or society. To make these spaces and maintain their viability is ongoing work. These elements, stemming from the radical history of studio art therapy, may now be a beacon for the future.

References

Harrison, A. (2009) Where Worlds Collide: The Studio and Beyond. In: *The Artist's Studio*. Waterfield, G. (Ed). Hogarth Arts, Tunbridge Wells.

Hogan, S. (2001) *Healing Arts: The History of Art Therapy*. Jessica Kingsley Publishers, London and Philadelphia.

Hogan, S. (2016) *Art Therapy Theories: A Critical Introduction*. Routledge, Oxen and New York.

Milner, J. (2009) Locating the Studio. In: *The Artist's Studio*. Waterfield, G. (Ed). Hogarth Arts, Tunbridge Wells.

Moon, C.H. (2002) *Studio Art Therapy: Cultivating the Artist Identity in the Art Therapist*. Jessica Kingsley Publishers, London and New York.

Moon, C.H. (2016) Open Studio Approach to Art Therapy. In: *The Wiley Handbook of Art Therapy*. Gussak, D. and Rosal, M.L. (Eds.). Wiley Blackwell, Chichester.

Omand, H. (2023) Drawing the Group: A Visual Exploration of a Therapeutic Space Online. In: *Art-Based Research in the Context of a Global Pandemic*. Seregina, U. and Van den Bossche, A. (Eds.). Routledge, New York and London.

Tipple, R. (2003) The Interpretation of Children's Artwork in a Paediatric Disability Setting. *Inscape: The Journal of the British Association of Art Therapists*. 8:2, 48–59.

Talwar, S. (2019) *Art Therapy for Social Justice: Radical Intersections*. Routledge, New York and London.

Part I
Frames of reference

1 Historical perspectives

Christopher Brown and Helen Omand

How to define art therapy in the UK has been a somewhat vexatious question from the beginning of its history, which makes it all the more difficult to pin down exactly when it started; Adrian Hill coined the term in 1942, but as Hogan points out in her history of art therapy (2001), art was being used as part of psychiatric treatment in the nineteenth century.

The reasons for this perplexing issue of definition lie in the specific social, cultural, and political contexts in the UK, in which the early pioneers developed their practice. There was a good deal of variety within this practice. From the latter half of the twentieth century, two divergent approaches emerged – one that emphasised making art as therapeutic, the other with art as mediator of the therapeutic relationship. In this chapter, we explore the tension within this apparent dialectic and consider its impact on the studio art therapy approach. We draw on existing published histories of art therapy and early art therapy texts, which tend to take different positions on this divide and emphasise the influence of either art or relationship on the profession's development (Waller, 1991; Hogan, 2001). Using original source material from art therapists who came after the early pioneers, we examine whether there was a 'psychoanalytic turn' away from studio practice during the development of the profession. In exploring this, it becomes clear that things are more complex, and practice more nuanced, as different ideas were integrated.

We acknowledge that we are writing from a UK perspective, and our focus is on what has happened to studio practice between the establishment of art therapy and the present day in this country. The context would be very different in other places. Gilroy and Hanna have this to say:

> The establishment of art therapy as a profession in various countries around the world requires attention to several different areas: to issues within the 'interest group' as it develops into a professional community; to the nature of mental health care and to relationships with allied professions; and to the broad social, political and cultural context of the country in question.
>
> (1998: 269)

DOI: 10.4324/9781003095606-3

The very notion of what art therapy is will vary from place to place and over time. Kapitan (2008), drawing on Vick's comparison of community studios in the US and Europe, points out many European studios did not consider themselves to be doing 'art therapy' at all, although they shared many of the same aims as US studio art therapists. Kapitan notes there are many 'not art therapy' endeavours happening globally: 'When a whole community embraces the idea of art as a healing technology and applies it to suit its own particular needs, a thousand permutations become possible on how art therapy may be defined' (2008: 2). When practice is on the innovative margins there are shades of grey between arts in health, community arts, healing arts, art as therapy and art therapy, which will shift according to history, context, and prevailing narrative.

Early influences

Early therapeutic art practices are complex to track (see Hogan, 2001; Waller, 1991), and we take up the story in the 1940s with the idea of making art as therapeutic in itself as epitomised by Adrian Hill and Edward Adamson. Both developed their practice in studios in hospital settings, working with tuberculosis and psychiatric patients respectively. Hill believed in the healing power of art, which took it beyond being an occupational activity, although that was often how it was presented to his patients and the medical establishment. Like Hill, Adamson was against any kind of interpretation or use of psychodynamic theory with patients. In his forward to Adamson's seminal book, *Art as Healing*, Anthony Stevens, a psychiatrist and Jungian analyst, conveys the essence of Adamson's approach:

> Intuitively he knew there to be a connection between creativity and healing, and he understood the importance of providing a sanctuary – a space, a *temenos*[1] – in which this connection could be made. His genius lies in his ability to create the *enabling space*.
>
> (Stevens, 1983 in Adamson, 1984: vii)

Here, the main ingredients for an art therapy studio are made clear – a 'safe haven' that offers an alternative to the constrictions and demands of a world that may feel unsafe or threatening and a therapist's mind that offers non-intrusive engagement.

The different idea of art therapy being part of a primarily psychotherapeutic treatment was there from the beginning in both the UK and the US with Irene Champernowne and Margaret Naumberg. In 1942, Champernowne established Withymead, a therapeutic community where use of a communal art studio was seen as an integral part of the work – the work being Jungian analysis – with an emphasis on a natural healing process. Naumberg developed her art therapy practice within a framework of Freudian psychoanalysis but preferred to allow the patient to discover symbolic meaning rather than offer interpretation (Hogan, 2001). The relationship between art therapy and psychoanalysis continued through the interests of pioneers such as Marion Milner and Ralph Pickford, who used art both in their personal analyses and subsequent work as psychotherapists.

However, Diane Waller, in her book, *Becoming a Profession: The History of Art Therapy in Britain 1940–82*, makes clear that the subsequent early pioneers in the UK tended to be artists, some involved in art education but all drawn in some way towards mental health settings and the art made there. These pioneer roles were often defined as 'artist' in order to avoid being aligned to occupational therapy and rehabilitation. She suggests that the role of artist was more attractive because of it having a higher status in the institutional hierarchy of mental hospitals (1991: 88/9).

As the emergent profession began to establish itself, the question of a more clearly defined role and identity became a preoccupation. Locating art in a medical world had its problems; art, and those who work with it, may be either distrusted or idealised by a medical establishment. Furthermore, the libertarian emphasis on subversion of psychiatric control and institutionalisation, which was prevalent in art therapy even before the antipsychiatry movement that emerged in the 1960s, did not sit well with the establishment. Eventually, there was a moving away from this position towards identification with more acceptable psychological models (Hogan, 2001). This move suggests a certain tension between the outsider position of artist and the need to fit into established medical paradigms.

During the 1950s and 1960s, when the aims of art therapy were being developed, Alexander Weatherson, a pioneer art therapist at Springfield Hospital, promoted the idea that art therapists should engage in exploration of both process *and* content. That is to say, being involved in the spontaneous making of the artwork through provision of a dedicated studio space, discussion about the artwork produced there, and interpretation of its content (Waller, 1991). Previously, these aspects tended to be separate, with the making process guided by the art therapist and the interpretation of content being the realm of psychiatrists or psychotherapists – seen as the higher function. In order to become more directly involved in the psychotherapy of patients in this way, some form of training became necessary (for a detailed account of the development of trainings, see Waller and James, 1984). There had always been those who had trained in either analytical psychology or psychoanalysis making use of art in therapy, but once formal training for art therapists began in academic settings during the 1970s, the need for theoretical underpinnings became pressing. The influence of these trainings on the direction that the profession took has to be acknowledged too. These reflected and perpetuated shifts in alliances; moving from arts education and social justice to teaching psychodynamic concepts, as tutors brought their own experiences of psychodynamic trainings to the courses.

Alongside the establishment of a professional organisation – British Association of Art Therapists in 1963 – and the development of training courses was the lobbying for recognised pay scales for art therapists during the 1980s. With these moves to become an autonomous profession came a desire to be seen as separate from occupational therapy and equated with those with higher status, such as psychology and speech therapy (Waller, 1991). It seems that this desire to be a discrete profession, and not merely an adjunct to another, impacted upon the so-called 'open group' model, which took place in large, open studios where the emphasis was on the patient's relationship to their artwork and less on their relationship with the therapist and other patients. The closing of many asylums in the 1980s and 1990s and the opening up of opportunities for art therapists in other care sectors (e.g. schools, day centres, social services, prisons) may well have contributed to a turning away from such open group models towards an interest in closed group and individual work, which in turn led to more encounters with transference phenomena and psychoanalytic ideas about how to manage them. Psychoanalytic trainings became desirable in order to fulfil individual desire for more knowledge and self-awareness, as well as a marker of status. However, this turning away from studios was only partial and there is anecdotal evidence that the practice of open studio groups continued to be a mainstay of practice in some settings.

From the 1970s to the present day, there have been numerous changes in the social, political, and economic climate that have affected the way art therapy practice has developed. Amongst these is the loss of spaces and places where studios could operate (see Wood, Chapter 3; Brown, Chapter 7), particularly within the NHS. While the importance of the physical environment is not to be underestimated, this loss has ultimately led to other innovations which have applied the ethos of studio practice to new spaces (see Lloyd and Usiskin, Chapter 8; Pratt, Chapter 11; Richardson, Chapter 18). Another change was the debate in the UK about what title practitioners should use, which emerged from negotiations with government bodies leading to State Registration in 1997 and the adoption of an equivalent protected title of 'art psychotherapist' to sit alongside that of 'art therapist'. It is not hard to imagine how status may also have played a part in the development of a potential two-tier terminology with its elitist implications, certainly there is plenty to be curious about in terms of how the idiosyncrasies of a particular social context shape a profession.

Reflecting on practice

This idea that there may have been a 'psychoanalytic turn' away from the studio, with its focus on the art, towards a practice of art therapy as a specialised form of psychotherapy appears in both Waller's history (1991), where art therapists are seen pragmatically adapting to changing circumstances, and in Hogan's history (2001), where art therapy as a profession is critiqued for moving too far from its libertarian artist roots. These narratives intrigued us. To investigate the possibility of a 'psychoanalytic turn', we approached a small number of art therapists working in the period 1970–2010. During this time frame, there was a period of growth in studio models followed by a period of decline from the mid-1980s onwards.

We asked these art therapists questions about their initial approach to the work; whether this was subsequently influenced by ideas from psychoanalytic psychotherapy and if this shift in framework affected practice; whether there was a consequent sense of turning away from studio art therapy; did it result in a focus on relational issues rather than the art; how did the setting for art therapy change over time during their career? The art therapists who responded reflected on their personal and professional histories and how these impacted on the development of their art therapy practice. All quotes given in the following pages are from personal communication in 2020 unless otherwise cited.

Several had experience early on of working in art studios in therapeutic communities. In the 1970s, Joy Schaverien, originally trained as a painter at the Slade, was employed as an art therapist at the Whitehouse therapeutic community in Brighton. Here, she worked as part of a multidisciplinary team. There was a large attic studio where she encouraged patients to create artworks using paint, clay, and performance art. The art therapy was an integral part of the dynamic of the whole group psychotherapy, community process. Here, she began to develop her understanding of the links between art therapy and psychotherapy. People also had access to the art room when she wasn't there and when she came in she would see what the patients had created and discuss the work with them. Occasionally, the walls of the studio had been painted with powerful therapeutic messages. It was both here, and in her subsequent work in a psychiatric hospital, that her interest in erotic transference began, as she sought to understand why patients might appear to be falling in love with their therapists. It seemed that the artwork played a role in this, and this led to her research. Her first writings during the 1980s investigated the role of the pictures in the transference–countertransference dynamic. Her research began, first as part of the MA at Birmingham College of Art and Design and culminated in a PhD and her book, *The Revealing Image: Analytical Art Psychotherapy in Theory and Practice*, published in 1991. The subtitle of this book reflects the attempt to develop a term that encompassed both the art and the analysis of the artworks. During the 1980s, she had become familiar with the strictly non-interpretative approach of Edward Adamson, who she knew personally from visiting his studio in Ashton, on the Rothschild Estate in Northamptonshire, on many occasions. She also encountered this approach while teaching on the training at St Albans, where she worked with Diana Halliday:

> This approach was very respectful of the image, but sometimes it seemed to miss out an element of mediating the disturbance in the person. That is what I felt was missing in the studio approach. Some patients need more; they need the therapist to speak; to give words that help to contain what emerges in the artwork.

Sometimes she thought talking could get in the way of the art making process, but at other times one could talk 'around' the artwork in a nuanced way that was different to interpretation. The understanding that the art making alone may not be enough informed her decision to train as an analyst with the Society of Analytical Psychology. She now works as a Jungian psychoanalyst and includes art materials in her room, as well as two chairs and a couch.

In another therapeutic community, the Henderson Hospital, the art therapist Jacky Mahony developed a number of different art therapy settings during the 1980s. She had already been exposed to group analytic ideas while working as a potter in the occupational therapy department at the Warneford Hospital and

undertook the introductory course at the Institute of Group Analysis before training as an art therapist in 1982. At the Henderson, she conducted an 'Art Work
Group' and an 'Art Psychotherapy Group' as well as other groups in the intensive
programme. In hindsight, she understood she was using a studio approach in the
art work group and that this seemed to be operating at a deeper level than the more
analytic art psychotherapy group 'which for this client group, was more threatening and stressful as well as verbally, content and transference focused'. In addition, she designed and set up another studio environment 'big enough for using a
wide range of media with different adjoining facilities, kiln room and discussion
area. It came to be used by residents and staff twenty-four hours a day' (Mahony,
2010: 225–226). In her next post working with psychiatric outpatients in the NHS
(1992–2003), she went on to do further group analytic training and developed
a model that used a longer time frame with more of a focus on art making than
talking. Doctoral research followed using visual arts methodologies to explore the
relationship between the therapist's personal art practice and its relationship to
such a group. Discussion centred around process rather than content, and clients
were encouraged to find parallels with their experiences in life outside the group.
The experience of making art in a supportive group led to 'an improved ability to
cope with them [symptoms] and with the associated feelings, including an acceptance that the difficulties were part of being human rather than an illness' (2010:
293). Mahony moreover argues that a studio approach allows for slower moving
serial craft processes to have an effect, often ignored in art psychotherapy. Craft
objects can critically comment on cultural, social and political contexts, offering
complicated visual interpretations. The therapist's art making makes visible the
complexities of reciprocal relationships and change over time.

Jane Dudley also worked at the Henderson – as an RMN Charge Nurse – and
this included time within art therapy groups as described by Jacky Mahony. She
had come from a medical model of psychiatry where medication or ECT was
usually the treatment of choice and patients had little say in their treatment. The
Henderson introduced her to

> a group analytic and democratic way of working with patients, who were
> called residents, where staff were required to explore and examine their
> selves as much as the residents were. She witnessed significant improvement
> without the use of medication. This enlightened approach ended, for her, the
> myth that as staff you were more expert and more 'sorted out' than the patient.

It also led her to train as an art therapist in 1987, feeling that the antipsychiatry
ethos within the profession at the time mirrored her work within the therapeutic
community. She found that the psychodynamic orientation of her training at Goldsmiths 'was not alien to me'. She subsequently worked in a well-established art
therapy studio within psychiatric services where

> [W]e emphasised the psychotherapeutic approach of accessing the uncon-
> scious and saw groups as a whole, where patients were empowered to have

'their say' and feel able to question and explore with each other, including the staff. We did not interpret but rather facilitated the client to find their own meaning.

This mirrors Naumberg's approach; in both cases there is an underpinning of ideas about the unconscious that come from psychoanalysis. Access to the unconscious mind that gives understanding of personal meaning in relational behaviour is the common ground between psychoanalysis and art therapy. Interpretation may or may not be part of technique in either. Dudley was instrumental in getting improved pay grades for art therapists during the Agenda for Change (1999) negotiations, but this may have led to demands on the profession to provide legitimacy through dominant establishment paradigms. There is a sense of regret perhaps when she says:

> I feel art therapy has lost its way in a sea of evidence with NICE guidelines, quantitative research and what seems to be an acceptance of medicalisation and treatments such as ECT. Art Therapy may have been accepted into the 'mainstream' but at what cost? I feel art therapy needs to realign itself with psychoanalysis and group analysis – it is a better home than the medical model of psychiatry, which sits with the sciences not the arts where art therapy/psychotherapy surely belongs.

Caroline Case trained on the course at St Albans in 1973–1974, when Edward Adamson was teaching there.

> The therapy group on the course was three hours in a studio with him and the whole course. He silently patrolled around us and offered very little comment. I remember 'what a pretty blue', over my shoulder. It is an experience which has stayed with me and one which I have tried to replicate as I feel it is sanctuary for the tired soul, not a known clinical condition but how people often arrive in therapy.

After training, Case worked with children and young people in the looked after system. Her experiences of 'trying to understand such distressed children's behaviour' led her to do an MA thesis on bereavement and later, in the early 1980s, to do the Psychoanalytic Observation Course at the Tavistock, leading her to train as a child psychotherapist in Edinburgh. She then practised both as an art therapist and as a child psychotherapist. In this way, psychoanalytic ideas were embraced because of a need to focus on the relationship in therapy. But this did not mean abandoning that version of a studio from her training experience, rather adapting it to whatever space was available. 'I find it difficult to separate the images and relational issues as it is all one'. The entirety of the non-verbal experience, that may be so present for art therapists working with children, may also be pronounced in the studio where there is less formalised explanation of the pictures; the gestures, the sounds and smells of materials, the glances and eye contact between the group and therapist, the play and movement around the room, all of which may be responded to by the therapist.

Robin Tipple developed his ideas about 'art making as *communication*' during his long career working in Learning Disability (LD), using studios, groups, and individual settings.

> I came to art therapy through working in a 'geriatric hospital' where I was employed as a mural artist, on Fridays the mural artists encouraged patients, who visited the studio where we worked, to use art materials. We also encouraged talk. So for me encouraging others to make art, looking at art and talk about art, was part of what I understood art therapy to be about. In training in 1983 we were given a crash course in psychodynamic theory, mostly Freud and Klein. I say 'crash course', because the training was then only for one year full-time.

Tipple subsequently worked in an LD Hospital where his interest in Kleinian and Marxist perspectives made him aware of 'my real difference in opinion to others' and 'a moment when I began to formulate, for myself, some kind of theoretical alliance in terms of practice'. He also undertook personal Kleinian psychoanalytic psychotherapy.

> In the main psychotherapy gave me confidence. I began to think in a more focussed way about relationship, about transference, about phantasy and the communication of feeling or affect. I probably became more critical of the art therapy literature. I stopped worrying about 'interpretations' – art therapists are always interpreting although they might pretend otherwise.

Crucially, this

> didn't diminish my interest in art and art making and in understanding this in relation to therapy. I made use of art history, semiotics, philosophy and other social and cultural studies, so I have broadened my approach to thinking in relation to art. This broadening of interest should in a way be understood as emerging from *research,* and research has shaped the profession.

Another art therapist who was interested in theory, Katherine Killick, has written extensively on studio-based art therapy for working with psychosis, where there is a loss of the symbolising function and fragmentation of the self. She summarises her approach in her introduction to the book *Art Therapy for Psychosis: Theory and Practice*, which she was commissioned to edit for The International Society for Psychological and Social Approaches to Psychosis Series:

> The need for a specifically structured psychotherapeutic relationship that respects and accommodates the extreme anxiety that lies at the core of psychotic states formed the subject of my own published work . . . The therapist's

understanding and acceptance of the patient's profound anxiety, and of the consequent use of the setting for self-protection, enables a particular form of primitive therapeutic alliance to develop. This exerts no pressure on the patient to engage prematurely in symbolic ways of relating, but it maintains a constant invitation to do so if and when he or she is able and willing.

(2017: 4)

Repeated experiences of this kind of studio art therapy setting may thus lead to relational engagement that allows images to be used for symbolic communication. In this way, the studio can become a 'place for the mind to heal' (Ibid.: 3). Killick acknowledges that 'Ideas from psychoanalysis gave me a theoretical framework which substantiated these principles'. Psychoanalytic thinking supported the significance that her approach gave to setting, art making and art objects. 'Attention to the images and the surrounding frame elements were central to my practice'. Indeed, the studio and the art made within it was of such importance that it led to a crisis.

The diminishing size of the available therapy space, the nature of the room and the absence of space for placing and storing images because it was shared with other professionals restricted the nature of the image making activities that were possible. This was a loss of such significance to me that I stopped practising as an art therapist.

She went on to train with the Society of Analytical Psychology and is now a Jungian analyst.

Diane Waller became interested in art therapy while studying at the Royal College of Art. She went on to work as an art therapist at the Paddington Centre for Psychotherapy, where there was a large art room with attached pottery and kiln.

I worked closely with the staff in the Day Centre who had a group analytic approach, with staff from the adult psychoanalytic department and also with the family and children area (where D.W. Winnicott had worked previously). Looking back, I would say I was influenced by Marxist art educators and critics like John Berger and thought mainly about art in a social/political context. I was not exactly suspicious but wary of individual psychoanalysis and wary about making interpretations from one specific theoretical position.

Waller initiated the training course at Goldsmiths in 1974 and undertook a group analytic training at the London Centre for Psychotherapy (LCP).

The director, Ilsa Seglow, was a graduate of the Frankfurt School and had combined her Marxist background with an approach to groups which was a combination of process sociology and group analysis. She had worked with S. H. Foulkes who together with Norbert Elias had been tutors at the Frankfurt School. Foulkes went on to develop group analytic psychotherapy at the

Institute for Group Analysis (IGA). I had chosen the London Centre from a sense that it was more radical/sociological than the IGA and was right in this, as pioneers such as Jafar Kareem, who founded Nafsiyat Intercultural Therapy Centre, were tutors and supervisors there. My supervisor was an artist himself and encouraged me to combine group analysis with art therapy. Whilst at Goldsmiths I was developing this model and colleagues also went to LCP and we began to use the 'interactive' model as part of the training. However, other colleagues who came to Goldsmiths had done a Jungian psychotherapy or an Objects Relations training, and Gerry McNeilly went to the IGA. So it was somewhat eclectic. Various psychotherapy models took different approaches to the artwork, but it is true to say that from around the early 1980s the relationship between the art therapist and the client became as important as the artwork itself. I felt that was a good thing.

Discussion

What becomes apparent from these accounts is that there was a lot of to and fro-ing between thinking about the art making process and psychoanalytic ideas. This suggests less of a 'psychoanalytic turn' and more a process of integration between ideas and approaches. It seems likely that the influence of personal therapy on practice enabled integration of ideas about psychology and art rather than divergence into an either or position – a move from the paranoid schizoid position to the depressive position perhaps (Klein, 1946). Less of a binary argument between studio and psychoanalytically informed practice, more the approach is led by an understanding of the needs of the client or group and influenced by further training and ideas.

Certainly, there was a need to pay attention to the transference and counter-transference, but this does not necessarily lead to interpretation along psychoanalytic lines. There is much nuance to what is said about the art in studios, and it is not so polarised as 'interpretation' versus 'silence'; in fact, these two positions seem to have been somewhat vilified by their opponents. In reality, art therapists and their clients talk 'about, around and into' the art (as Schaverien told us), with an emphasis on the client's own understanding of their work. A nuanced example of this is Jacky Mahony's discussions about the process of making and the parallels with life outside of the group for clients. In this regard, the talking about art may depend upon the context in which the frame sits, such as art psychotherapist, studio manager, group worker, or educationalist for example. There was a process of adaptation according to the needs dictated by the context, which in turn leads to adaptation of the frame. We can see the influence of schools of thought and further training (social and political as well as psychoanalytic), whilst the studio frame retains its essence; a certain freedom for the client in how the space is used, more time for art making processes to develop and the privileging of the client's own understanding of their art.

Radical ideas about groups were certainly an influence on art therapists working in studios in therapeutic communities, such as Jane Dudley and Jacky Mahony.

The political leanings of this can't be underestimated. Socialism was also part of the context of art therapy as it developed and both Tipple and Waller acknowledged an interest in Marxism. Waller said,

> I realise I am still very much influenced by the socio-political thinking of the Frankfurt School, Elias and process sociology, and by thinking about art in that context – about art's role in society as well as its meaning to the individual.

The Institute for Social Research was founded in Germany in 1924 to provide a critical theory of Marxism; the people and ideas associated with it became known as the Frankfurt School. Their ideas permeated post-war thinking and the development of critical theory in relation to society, culture, and media. Their goal was the radical transformation of society.

Adorno, one of their leading proponents, formulated the idea of a 'culture industry' in which culture was a key instrument of political and social control. Another was Marcuse, whose ideas were seen as a rejection of forms of oppression and domination, which captured the revolutionary mood of the 1960s (Jeffries, 2017). The school's leading contemporary figure, Habermas, developed their model of critical theory into and beyond post-modernism. He believed 'that through rational communication we can overcome our biases, our egocentric and ethnographic perspectives, come to a consensus or community of reason' (Jeffries, 2017: 358). These ideas influenced art therapists who were working with the disenfranchised and framed their work in a sociopolitical context. For example, in the accounts of Dudley, Tipple, and Waller, who worked with groups, we can see the impact of social as well as psychological influences. The continued relevance of social and psychoanalytical groups' thinking for art therapy practice today in a post pandemic world is evident, as echoed in a recent videoconference presentation of a paper by Christopher Bollas (2021), who was involved in the social justice movement in the US, before he came to the UK to train as a psychoanalyst in the 1970s. In an examination of the large group we call a nation (referring to the US), he highlights psychotic processes that threaten to dismantle the structures of group conscience necessary to contain sociopathic behaviour and which could lead to the collapse of civilisation. He advocates public discussion to engage with the psychopathologies of the large group, using people skilled in group relations, to 'free the group to come to more considered and sane solutions'.

It is possible to trace ideas about the social, political, and economic contexts that have influenced the frame(s) within which art therapy has been, and is, practiced. From the 'enlightenment', itself seeped in colonial history, through libertarianism to the utopias of the 1960s, runs a complex and sometimes problematic thread, a desire to liberate the downtrodden and dispossessed, and a wish for equality. At the same time, repressive forces in society work to maintain 'our enslavement within the totality of capitalist social relations' (Jeffries, 2017: 231). The tension between these two forces is felt throughout contemporary society and infuses art therapy's history. We can link this to early studio art therapists embracing an antipsychiatry position to provide a sanctuary in the midst of oppressive medical practices; the wish to create a space apart from the inequalities of society, and yet by our role as art therapists we are part of the hierarchical system we struggle against.

Recent history shows the impact of free market economies and managerialism on the legitimisation of services provided by the NHS and local authorities. Austerity measures have resulted in a cutting of services, particularly in community services for adults and children's services that include art therapy. The need for evidence-based interventions has led to alignments with developments in neuroscience and psychology such as 'mentalization'. Another 'turn' the profession seemed to take was away from an appreciation of unconscious processes, in the individual, groups, and society, towards frameworks that offer quick solutions to complex problems (Dalal, 2018). In this way, we can see a swing away from the psychoanalytic, with psycho-educational, mindfulness, compassion-focussed, and cognitive analytic therapies emerging as other influences on practice (BAAT, 2020). The swing of the free market also tends to be by its nature towards individualism and away from the sociopolitical emphasis of the power of groups, a balance readdressed by many of the chapters to follow. It is in this climate that the book investigates both the survival of studio art therapy as a core method and its development in contemporary settings.

Note

1   'Temenos: temple enclosure or court in ancient Greece: a sacred precinct' *Merriam-Webster.com Dictionary*, Merriam-Webster, www.merriam-webster.com/dictionary/temenos. Accessed 29 March 2020.

References

Adamson, E. (1984) *Art as Healing*. Coventure, London.

Bollas, C. (2021) Civilization and the Discontented. In: *Psychoanalysis and Covidian Life: Common Distress, Individual Experience*. Levine, H.B. and Staal, A. (Eds.). Phoenix Publishing House. Community West videoconference presentation by Christopher Bollas recorded on 8 August 2020.

British Association of Art Therapists (2020) What Is Art Therapy? www.baat.org/about-art-therapy (Accessed 12 April 2020).

Dalal, F. (2018) *CBT: The Cognitive Behavioural Tsunami. Managerialism, Politics and the Corruptions of Science*. Routledge, Abingdon, Oxon.

Department of Health. (1999) *Agenda for Change – Modernising the NHS Pay System. Health Service Circular HSC 1999/035*. Department of Health, London. www.dh.gov.uk/en/Publicationsandstatistics/Lettersandcirculars/Healthservicecirculars/DH_4003632.

Gilroy, A. and Hanna, M. (1998) Conflict and Culture: An Australian Perspective. In: *Tapestry of Cultural Issues in Art Therapy*. Hiscox, A. and Calisch, A. (Eds.). Jessica Kingsley Publishers, London.

Hogan, S. (2001) *Healing Arts: The History of Art Therapy*. Jessica Kingsley Publishers, London.

Jeffries, S. (2017) *Grand Hotel Abyss: The Lives of the Frankfurt School*. Verso, London.

Kapitan, L. (2008) "Not Art Therapy": Revisiting the Therapeutic Studio in the Narrative of the Profession. *Art Therapy*. 25:1, 2–3.

Killick, K. (Ed.) (2017) *Art Therapy for Psychosis: Theory and Practice*. Routledge, Abingdon, Oxon.

Klein, M. (1946) 'Notes on Some Schizoid Mechanisms' in *The Writings of Melanie Klein*, vol. 3, pp. 1–24. Vintage, London.

Mahony, J. (2010) *Reunion of Broken Parts'(Arabic al-jabr) – A Therapist's Personal Art Practice and Its Relationship to an NHS Outpatient Art Psychotherapy Group: An Exploration Through Visual Arts and Crafts Practice*. PhD thesis, Goldsmiths, University of London.

Schaverien, J. (1991) *The Revealing Image: Analytical Art Psychotherapy in Theory and Practice*. Routledge, London, New York (Current Edition Published by Jessica Kingsley (1999 & 2009).

Waller, D. (1991) *Becoming a Profession: The History of Art Therapy in Britain, 1940–82*. Routledge, London.

Waller, D. and James, K. (1984) Training in Art Therapy. In: *Art as Therapy*. Dalley, T. (Ed.). Tavistock Publications, London.

2 Literature review

Helen Omand and Dalaila Bumanglag

This chapter follows the twists and turns of studio practice in art therapy literature and draws out prevalent themes, roughly chronologically, from a rich body of literature, not all of which could be included. It focuses on UK practice with adults with a limited selection of US literature as a counterpoint.

What do we think we mean by studio art therapy?

If we take recent UK introductory guides to art therapy as a barometer, studio art therapy is either referred to historically, exemplified by Hill and Adamson in the 1940s, or, as practiced today, commonly framed as a genre of art therapy groups (Case and Dalley, 2014; Edwards, 2014). *Art studio groups, studio approach, open studio, open art therapy groups,* and *studio-based open groups* are used variously to describe some of the same principles of approach (Case and Dalley, 2014; Edwards, 2014, Hogan, 2014, 2015). There is clearly a set of collectively held ideas about this type of art therapy. So, what *is* it, according to this literature?

Most authors highlight the particular boundaries of the studio approach with agreement that these boundaries differ from conventional psychoanalytically informed groups. Clients work individually at their own pace and may choose to get up and wander around the room in search of inspiration, conversation, or simply for a break. The art therapist may circulate around the group, stopping to discuss pictures individually, while others carry on making art. There is often no particular structure for art making or talking, and clients may walk in and out of the room within the agreed time frame with no pressure to stay in the group. Words like 'free', 'open', 'relaxed', and 'non-rigid' appear in these descriptions and convey something of the atmosphere, contrasting with analytically based art therapy group boundaries. Hogan (2014) points out a studio group may feel more like collection of individuals, and membership being open or closed will affect the extent to which sessions feel consistent and more 'group-like'. Generally, there is less emphasis on analysing group processes and interactions. For example, in any group there will be rivalries for the attention of the art therapist, but group dynamics are not usually thought to be the focus in studio art therapy (Schaverien, 1991; Hogan, 2014).

DOI: 10.4324/9781003095606-4

Instead, the focus is the art making process itself and there is broad agreement that treatment of the art is different in studio art therapy. Easels and individual work areas may evoke the dedicated space of an artist's studio and along with it perhaps the option to use a wider range of materials such as oil paints, plaster, or canvases for example and to make a mess. Other differences are highlighted in the lack of expectation for the client to talk about their work. The focus on ongoing art processes means more time and attention can be spent by the artist developing the work. Schaverien describes:

> This type of art therapy group enables a very deep level of self-exploration through the pictures. Often this is far deeper than in groups where the dynamics and the transference are interpreted. There is freedom to explore where the image leads without obligation to show the picture.
>
> (1991: 4)

This foregrounding of the image-making process over time is emphasised by Hogan (2014) as a strength of studio art therapy. She points out, this addresses some of the problems with conventional art therapy groups identified by Skaife and Huet (1998), when new artworks are made every session, bringing a surplus of material but with no opportunity of developing the image further.

Case and Dalley (2014) comment on a more recent resurgence in studio ways of working, but this literature generally does not expand on what the framework of studio art therapy allows or hinders, its suitability or not for different client groups, how the studio approach has been developed recently or where it is located now in the UK.

In the US, studio approaches are well developed as a diverse set of practices with an ethos distinct from much of mainstream art therapy (Allen, 2016; Moon, 2016; Vick, 2016). Junge writes:

> The Studio Art approach is a community art studio in which the art therapist as an artist acts as a *facilitator* of art media and processes, rather than as a *doctor* of a patient with a mental illness or dysfunction.
>
> (2010: 258 italics in original)

Moon (2016) also identifies a non-clinical approach aligned with health rather than an illness model, which reorientates identity from service user to artist/ maker, emphasising a levelled power dynamic, communality, and a democratic approach. She notices art studios in the US may have something of an egalitarian ideology and a politically and ethically informed stance. Moon characterises an open studio approach as art based and draws attention to the term 'open', suggesting it may refer to boundaries, non-directive working, client population, or the therapist's attitude of transparency. She suggests attendance can be more casual through word of mouth or drop in within a community making it accessible for those who would not access conventional therapy.

The UK pioneers: the enabling space and the power of expression

An early account of a therapeutic studio is from artist Adrian Hill, whose personal experience of painting while ill with tuberculosis led him to found a studio in a sanatorium to help other patients do the same. Hill, often taking a teacherly approach, saw art as healing rather than just diversionary, either by catharsis to free up the patient from difficult feelings or by distraction from 'morbid introspection' (Hill, 1945: 33 in Waller, 1991).

Adamson worked with Hill and set up his own studio at Netherne Hospital in 1946. In Adamson's view the art was a 'window' onto the patient's psyche and therein lay its potential for healing (Adamson, 1984). Adamson was strictly non-interpretive and believed the patient held 'the only true meaning of a work' – to interpret risked the therapist finding only an obliging mirror of their own psychological orientation (1984: 7). To begin with, research was undertaken by the psychiatrists Cunningham Dax and Reitman who discussed paintings done in the studio with their patients, later Adamson worked without their input. Adamson's straightforward writing style is absent of any jargon, always seeing the person rather than the diagnosis, pointing out that medical terminology distances the patient 'like a specimen' (Ibid.).

In parallel, Jungian analyst Irene Champernowne set up Withymead, the influential therapeutic community, which revolved around a studio open to patients and staff alike and staffed by an art therapist. Champernowne describes an experience of using the studio; 'The peace and sincerity of the painting class drew it [a picture] out of me despite the storm and stress of outer life, and emphasised for me the value of this atmosphere created in the art rooms with such fertilising presiding spirits as the art therapists.' (Champernowne, cited in Hogan, 2001: 259). However, it was not the art therapist's role to interpret paintings. Lyddiatt (1971), influenced by her own analysis at Withymead, worked in a psychiatric hospital and emphasised the particular quality of being that a studio promotes: 'Often what is desirable for an art department is reminiscent of the quiet pondering of adults who in solitude play in streams and wander on the seashore' (1971: 14). Lyddiatt describes spontaneous painting that 'works back' on the artist. 'This 'thing' moves and changes us, provided we feel and value it and cease to demand reasons' (1971: 13). The 'demanding reasons' points, like Adamson, to a suspicion of overzealous psychiatric or psychoanalytic interpretation.

Growing tensions: libertarianism, antipsychiatry, and psychoanalysis

Tensions have often centred around the thorny matter of interpretation of images. The non-interventionist stance of early practitioners is in contrast to later ideas, which brought art and interpretation together in psychoanalytically informed art therapy (see Schaverien, 1991). In her historical account, Hogan (2001) argues that the various practices of pioneer artists of the 1950s and 1960s (she lists Glass,

Henzell, Weatherson and Simon), carried an egalitarian ethos of empowerment and subversion of psychiatric control, in contrast to growing psychoanalytic influences that she holds up as oppressively power infused. As studio practice grew, the scarcity of contemporary published literature makes it hard to track the development of the non-interpretative stance. So, what were art therapists actually saying, or not saying, about the art in their studios?

An insight is provided by a 1978 exhibition catalogue of 'The Inner Eye', an exhibition of patients' artwork submitted by art therapists, held at the Museum of Modern Art Oxford. The catalogue reveals descriptions by around twenty art therapists of their approaches, mainly in hospitals, with some therapeutic communities and special educational needs schools. Taken as a barometer, a glance through shows the popularity of ideas from early studio practice: the studio atmosphere required 'a quality of quiet' (Cohen: 39) and art therapists see their role as non-clinical, 'a helper or co-worker', a 'catalyst and facilitator rather than being an instructor or analyst' (Nowell-Hall: 39–40), 'offering oneself in an undogmatic way' (Walker: 37). Bostock says: 'If interpretations are made it is important that they are made by the creators of the work themselves' (Bostock: 36). Several art therapists describe encouraging clients to interpret their own work, the art, and the 'therapy' being brought together into the studio space. There is however 'understanding and respect for what is left unsaid' and for clients who prefer not to talk about the work (Cantwell: 38). The influence of antipsychiatry thinking is evident. Holtom writes 'The art therapy department in a psychiatric hospital is often an asylum within an asylum. That is to say it is a refuge from the depersonalising manoeuvres of a large institution and its agents' (Holtom: 40). New shoots of psychodynamic thinking are also present in some descriptions, with talk of 'the therapeutic relationship' (Goldsmith: 39) and 'reintegration of the personality' (Griffith: 41) but with the emphasis on the client's agency to use the space and relationship to the extent they chose.

Henzell, working at Napsbury Hospital with R.D. Laing in the 1960s in the height of the antipsychiatry movement, describes the approach in his studio: 'I did not allow the language or habits of orthodox psychotherapeutic practice to distract patients from the play of imagination made possible by the materials' (1997: 181). However, although he criticises 'the therapist's professional need to translate this imagining into Freudian, Jungian, Kleinian or other such schema', he does acknowledge that such theories can function usefully when they meet the image in its own right (Ibid.). Unlike Adamson who was notoriously silent, Henzell's case vignette describes many conversations about his patient's art that 'grew out of their style and content' (1997: 182). Crucially, the emphasis was on letting the patient's meaning of their art develop rather than making a psychoanalytic interpretation. Henzell names the increasing tension in the 1960s and 1970s as art therapy developed, 'the pragmatism required in obtaining a necessary professional recognition has perhaps led art therapy into a somewhat contradictory position, a situation which has often forced its practitioners to choose between the art or therapy aspects of their craft' (1978: 33).

In 1984, as if to challenge Adamson's *Art as Healing*, another book appeared on the scene, *Art as Therapy*, which brought together art and psychotherapy. Editor Dalley emphasised the picture's symbolic meaning within the therapeutic relationship: 'The drawing process itself is not the sole therapeutic agent. Like dreams, pictures have little meaning in isolation' (1984: xiii). By the early 1990s, Woddis suggests the debate was intensifying between the 'Healing Arts' and psychodynamic art psychotherapy (1993: 27).

> The 'open door' arrangement which has prevailed in many hospitals since the 1940s in which the art room is seen as a haven in a hostile environment, where music might be playing and tea may be served and where all are welcome for as long or short a time as they can tolerate the atmosphere, will not be seen as a serious form of treatment but rather a diversionary activity and consequently more difficult to justify.
>
> (Woddis, 1993: 30)

An alternative history: US studio art therapy development

Moon proposes the history of open studios in the US differs from mainstream institutional and psychodynamic developments. However, unlike the UK, it is rooted in community practice: 'It is the story of how the process of art-making has been used for therapeutic aims, particularly within the context of community' (2016: 112). Wix regards the history of art therapy studios as a neglected but key aspect to the profession's beginnings, whose artistic roots are often lost in officially sanctioned, 'authoritative' histories (2010: 178). Wix (2010) points out that as well as Florence Cane and Edith Kramer's contributions to art as therapy, unsung artists like Mary Huntoon pioneered approaches from the 1930s, which grounded art in health not pathology. Junge (2010), Moon (2016) and Stepney (2019) point out the previously unacknowledged contribution of art therapists of colour to the artistic foundation of the profession; for example, Georgette Powell, Cliff Joseph, Lucile Venture, and Charles Anderson engaged in community approaches and activist arts promoting diversity, social justice and advocacy.

Junge (2010) suggests it wasn't until the 1990s that community studios became recognised as a particular approach within US art therapy. Certainly, literature gains momentum: Allen (1992) warns of 'clinification' and calls for art therapists to make art, in part to stay in touch with the uncertainty of therapeutic work rather than taking on the mantel of interpreter or clinical expert. Other accounts include Allen's (1995) gallery studio, McGraw's (1995) hospital-based studio (founded in 1967) and McNiff's (1995) spiritual approach. Moon's imaginative and seminal book *Studio Art Therapy: Cultivating the Artist Identity in the Art Therapist* proposes 'a model of art therapy wherein the products and processes of art constitute the core of the work rather than serving as the basis for theoretical adaptations from other disciplines' (2002: 20). Like in the UK, a split is perceived with mainstream art therapy practice (Malchiodi, 1995; Allen, 1992, 1995), although with hindsight viewed as a false dichotomy (Potash et al., 2016, see also Kapitan, Chapter 4, Andrus, Chapter 17).

Looking back and moving on: UK writing on the lost asylum studio

Since Adamson and Lyddiatt's contributions, detailed accounts of studios have been written retrospectively (e.g. Brown, 2014; Charlton, 1984; Goldsmith, 2006; Henzell, 1997; Wood, 1997, 2000). There is the sense of looking back on a bygone age of asylum studios and much of this writing sees what is valuable about a lost way of working, under-represented in the literature at the time. From these accounts an idea of the archetypal hospital studio emerges – spacious, accommodating, with paint-covered tables inviting mess. Some residents had their own workspaces they could return to, often over years, to develop their art practice, sometimes stuffed with books and bric-a-brac gathering dust amongst stacks of old artworks. All in stark contrast to the bare clinical spaces and potentially oppressive regimes in the wider hospital environment. Charlton comments on the effect of such a space on patients:

> By contrast to the ward the art room is a place where residents can make their own choices, within the sphere of creative activity, without fear of the consequences. Implicit in the art making process is permission to get messy, to experiment, to ponder or to invent.
>
> (1984: 185)

Charlton emphasises the promotion of agency, or free choice, to combat the disempowering effects of institutionalisation for incarcerated long-stay residents. Charlton is thinking about her studio work rather differently here, in that she is looking beyond the spontaneous Jungian dialogue with self to search for other therapeutic elements. Charlton adapted studio work to the needs of her patient groups, and she starts to frame some of her work in the benefits that group interactions can bring. For example, patients in her studio make tea for one another and look after materials; a mural painting group elicits a need for negotiation, all inviting the experience of self in relation to others (1984).

Saotome's (1998) research specifically examines the role of group practice in the last remaining asylum studios in the early 1990s. She argues that even traditional studio-based open groups foster an ethos of containment and commonality in a social context: 'The concept of 'group', though not declared the 'medium' of treatment, was surely evident and of therapeutic value to residents attending sessions' (1998: 159). Her study found practices varied, ranging from traditional studio groups open to all patients, to closed membership groups and theme-based sessions, yet these nonetheless encompassed similarities in that most operated on an individually focused basis but within a group setting. Her own approach combined group thinking with an informality of approach; tea and coffee were served, there was no obligation to show pictures, and ongoing art processes were common.

Killick (2000), Charlton (1984) and Goldsmith (2006) describe their studio approaches where the consistent space, combined with thoughtful and flexible boundaries, facilitated patients' gradual engagement so that they could develop at their own pace; it could take weeks or months to start making artwork, something perhaps not possible in today's tendency for short-term art therapy sessions. Being able to decide when to engage, and in what manner, fosters agency from the very beginning of the encounter (see also Cavaliero, Chapter 13), as does the studio environment itself which tangibly invites the patient to be active themselves in the therapy (Wood, 2000).

Goldsmith (2006) describes the move from hospital to a community studio and the difficulties in the changed time boundaries. Goldsmith points out, no longer could a patient drift in through an open door from the hospital grounds when the moment felt right, but rather they must navigate, very possibly in a psychotic state of mind, the uncertainty of public encounters; the bus, the waiting room, their own ambivalence, and some patients could not manage this. Saotome (1998) suggests that there was a general trend away from studio-based open groups towards more formalised models with fixed time boundaries and increased awareness of group dynamics in a framework of group analysis, and she highlights the influence of art therapy trainings from the early 1970s on this.

Wood (2000: 40) calls for a re-evaluation of the role of studios and amongst many convincing arguments emphasises the quality of absorption that studios promote; 'Absorption is the opposite of alienation', as well as tracing psychodynamic ideas around containment as conceptualised in relation to studio practice. She sets out the complexity of the social, political, and economic context surrounding the asylum closures and the enthusiastic take-up of psychodynamic ideas, arguing strongly that the latter should not mean studios are no longer needed; 'there is no reason why greater theoretical clarity cannot encompass a studio-based practice', and she is critical of the idea art therapists can sustain work in healthcare without the containment of a thought-out permanent space (2000: 48).

Into the twenty-first century: the development of UK and US studio practice

Despite closure of many asylums, inpatient work influenced by studio practices continued in psychiatric hospitals in the UK, developing according to the therapist's theoretical orientations. Luzzatto (1997) developed a studio approach suggesting that the therapist can consider group dynamics within an open session format, the flexibility of which means patients can use aspects of the space, the art, the therapist, and the group to a lesser or greater extent. Killick contributes a body of work (see her contribution to Brown and Omand, Chapter 1), drawing on psychoanalytic ideas about containment, for example Bick (1968), to suggest that the concrete nature of the studio space can facilitate interactions that over time can lead to symbolisation and emergence of a sense of self (Killick, 2000). Building on Killick's work, Deco (1998) uses Winnicott's theories to conceptualise her ward-based studio group as a transitional space. As her chapter title 'Return to the open studio group: art therapy groups in acute psychiatry' suggests, she proposes a reappraisal of studio models. Brown (2008) also examines the role of the setting in establishing therapeutic relationship and draws on Winnicott's (1965) writing on the facilitating environment, to develop the idea of the studio as a maternal function. Bonneau (2017) continues this line of thinking, referencing Killick and drawing on an existential, phenomenological, and psychodynamic approach. He emphasises the spatiality and corporeality of the studio space itself, where at first interactions are held in physical objects and the setting rather than in the internal worlds of therapist and client.

Other explorations of studio practice in the UK include the therapist's art making. Marshall-Tierney (2014) describes the therapist's art making as having a maternal function in his acute inpatient studio group. Mahony (2011) notes the benefits of ongoing craft processes in her outpatient studio group and examines her own artwork in relation to the group's to gain perspectives on shifting group dynamics (2011). Authors agree this practice can lessen clinical power dynamics, building on Greenwood and Layton's (1987) side-by-side approach (see also Omand and McMahon, Chapter 12). Something of an egalitarian influence continues with the therapist as artist, paralleling US literature, while points of difference from the US lie in the influence of psychodynamic and group analytic thinking in the UK.

Art therapists consider studios in other political contexts. Kalmanowitz and Lloyd (1997) brought the conceptual framework of 'The Portable Studio' to places of political conflict and develop this further in relation to ideas of home as a place in the mind (Kalmanowitz and Lloyd, 2005). Lloyd and Usiskin (2020) build on this work with migrants on the UK–France border, using 'The Community Table' concept. They note a necessary awareness of cultural imperialism and Eurocentricity and advocate looking beyond traditional art materials and practices to relevant arts-based practices that support social action and crisis intervention. Martyn (2019) and Kaczynski (2020) portray the work of The New Art Studio, a therapeutic studio for asylum seekers and refugees in London, with a particular focus by Martyn on the role of exhibiting. Omand (2022) describes a community studio for adults experiencing enduring mental health difficulties, where artworks function as political protest about harsh economic 'austerity' policies in the UK and embody a radical ethos for the group.

A growing area of development in the US is a socially informed emphasis on community empowerment, which recognises the community art studio as having potential for ethically informed social action (Kapitan, 2008). Although social justice agendas are not fundamental in an open studio approach, the collective, communal aspects of the work make it hard to ignore participants' external realities that are subject to social and political injustices and the 'links between individual and social change' (Moon, 2016: 118), (see also Armstrong, Chapter 9).

Block, Harris and Laing (2005) report on an open studio as a model of social action in response to the needs of at-risk youth. Adults making art alongside young people models and inspires creative risk-taking and contributes to effectiveness. Moon and Shuman's open studio creates an accessible community space for those 'with and without social stigma' (2013: 194), including people who may be marginalised because of their mental or physical health, homelessness or substance misuse. An egalitarian environment is encouraged through the common ground of 'art and culture making' and emphasis on 'radical inclusivity, stigma reduction, collective community building and emancipatory intent' (2013: 199). The authors describe how power imbalances, if never eliminated, are reduced wherever possible. Malis suggests a non-clinical studio environment enabled adults with mental illness to gain a sense of their own artistic identity and 're-experience themselves outside the confines of stigma' (2017: 6). Allen (2008) notes a democratic idea of art for all, often aiming to mix marginalised groups with the mainstream, where cultural activism can grow, including critiques of mainstream US material culture.

The use of galleries and exhibitions allow individuals to reframe their identities as artists and meet the wider community to exhibit, sell artwork, or challenge stigma to bring about social change (Thompson, 2009; Vick, 2016; Morris and Willis-Rauch, 2014; see also Armstrong, Chapter 9; Andrus, Chapter 17). Vick writes about a studio for artists with disabilities, with a social agenda that aims to shift negative social perceptions of 'disabled' and 'limited', to participants being seen as 'thriving artists' (2016: 837). Miller (2020) brings ideas from the Disability Art movement to studio exhibition practice, critiquing concepts of 'normalisation'. Ethics and power imbalances are pressing matters for art therapists working outside of existing institutional guidelines and Moon (2016) has emphasised the need for ethically informed community consultation. Timm-Bottos and Rosemary (2015) similarly highlight the importance for students to acquire skills that advocate for collaborative practices by using a 'third space' storefront classroom doubling as a community art studio, also explored by Franklin, Rothaus and Schpok (2006).

Increasingly, art therapists are also responding to the need for evaluative evidence-based research on studio practice. Kaimal et al. (2017) compare art therapist-facilitated open studio sessions and colouring-in exercises for adults. Both resulted in reduced stress and negative affect, yet the open studio sessions demonstrated significant improvements in self-efficacy, self-perceptions of creativity and positive mood. In the UK, Allan et al. investigate the benefits of a recovery-based art therapy group for adults with severe mental health needs. The physical setting of a community studio was an important factor for members, which enabled a 'stronger sense of artistic identity' (2015: 16). Nolan (2019) examines the mechanisms that influence therapeutic change in community studios and calls for the field of art therapy to broaden its scope of practice outside of clinical environments. Kapitan notices that studios in community-based settings are well positioned to be 'incubators for new ideas' (2008: 2) and are ideally placed for participatory action research, which finds new and democratic ways of collectively generating research, by groups who have been marginalised by the mainstream. New knowledge can then be brought to the field of art therapy overall.

This review has brought together some of the body of literature on what has become known as studio art therapy, now more than ever a diverse set of practices across settings, encompassing the development of different theoretical orientations. It has traced threads of influence such as social change and psychodynamic thinking through the decades of its practice in inpatient settings and beyond. Much of recent US literature focuses on community empowerment and makes a strong argument for the collaborative creation of open studios as innovative and flexible spaces where art is at the centre. The following chapters of the book continue to develop these different threads in the rich and complex tapestry that makes up studio practice today.

References

Adamson, E. (1984) *Art as Healing*. London: Coventure.

Allan, J., Barford, H., Horwood, F., Stevens, J. and Tanti, G. (2015) ATIC: Developing a recovery-based art therapy practice. *International Journal of Art Therapy*. 20:1. pp. 14–27.

Allen, P.B. (1992) Artist-in-residence: An alternative to "Clinification" for art therapists. *Art Therapy*. 9:1. pp. 22–29.

Allen, P.B. (1995) Coyote comes in from the cold: The evolution of the open studio concept. *Art Therapy*. 12:3. pp. 161–166.

Allen, P.B. (2008) Commentary on community-based art studios: Underlying principles. *Art Therapy*. 25:1. pp. 11–12.

Allen, P.B. (2016) Art making as spiritual path: The open studio process as a way to practice art therapy. In: Rubin, J.A. (ed.) *Approaches to Art Therapy: Theory and Technique* (3rd ed.). London: Routledge. pp. 271–285.

Bick, E. (1968) The experience of the skin in early object relations. *International Journal of Psycho-Analysis*. 49. pp. 484–486.

Block, D., Harris, T. and Laing, S. (2005) Open studio process as a model of social action: A program for at-risk youth. *Art Therapy*. 22:1. pp. 32–38.

Bonneau, J. (2017) The structured studio setting: An ontological dimension in art psychotherapy with psychosis using the concept of body image as structuring function. In: Killick, K. (ed.) *Art Therapy for Psychosis: Theory and Practice*. Oxon: Routledge. pp. 90–114.

Bostock, D. (1978) Catalogue. In: *The Inner Eye*. Elliot, D. (Ed.). Oxford: Museum of Modern Art. pp 15–41.

Brown, C. (2008) Very toxic – handle with care. Some aspects of the maternal function in art therapy. *Inscape*. 13:1. pp. 13–24.

Brown, C. (2014) The lost studio: "You don't know what you've got till it's gone." *ATOL: Art Therapy OnLine*. 5:1. https://journals.gold.ac.uk/index.php/atol/article/view/345/375.

Cantwell, M. (1978) Catalogue. In: *The Inner Eye*. Elliot, D. (Ed.). Oxford: Museum of Modern Art. pp. 35–41.

Case, C. and Dalley, T. (2014) *Handbook of Art Therapy* (3rd ed.). London: Routledge.

Charlton, D. (1984) Art therapy with long stay residents of psychiatric hospitals. In: Dalley, T. (ed.) *Art as Therapy. An Introduction to the Use of Art as a Therapeutic Technique*. London, New York: Routledge. pp. 173–190.

Cohen, M. (1978) Catalogue. In: *The Inner Eye*. Elliot, D. (Ed.). Oxford: Museum of Modern Art. pp. 35–41.

Dalley, T. (1984) Introduction. In: Dalley, T. (ed.) *Art as Therapy. An Introduction to the Use of Art as a Therapeutic Technique*. London, New York: Routledge. pp. xi–xxviii.

Deco, S. (1998) Return to the open studio group: Art therapy groups in acute psychiatry. In: Huet, V. and Skaife, S. (eds.) *Art Psychotherapy Groups: Between Pictures and Words*. Hove: Routledge. pp. 88–108.

Edwards, D. (2014) *Art Therapy* (2nd ed.). London: Sage.

Franklin, M., Rothaus, M.E. and Schpok, K. (2006) Unity in diversity: Communal pluralism in the art studio and the classroom. In: Kaplan, F. (ed.) *Art Therapy and Social Action*. London: Jessica Kingsley. pp. 213–230.

Goldsmith, A. (1978) Catalogue. In: *The Inner Eye*. Elliot, D. (Ed.). Oxford: Museum of Modern Art. pp. 35–41.

Goldsmith, A. (2006) The art therapy room. In: Case, C. and Dalley, T. (eds.) *Handbook of Art Therapy* (2nd ed.). London: Routledge. pp. 60–83.

Greenwood, H. and Layton, G. (1987) An outpatient art therapy group. *Inscape*, Summer. pp. 12–19.

Griffith, S. (1978) Catalogue. In: *The Inner Eye*. Elliot, D. (Ed.). Oxford: Museum of Modern Art. pp. 35–41.

Henzell, J. (1978) Art and psychopathology: A history of its study and applications. In: *The Inner Eye*. Elliot, D. (Ed.). Oxford: Museum of Modern Art.

Henzell, J. (1997) Art, madness and anti-psychiatry: A memoir. In: Killick, K. and Shaverien, J. (eds.) *Art, Psychotherapy and Psychosis*. London: Routledge. pp. 176–197.

Hogan, S. (2001) *The Healing Arts: The History of Art Therapy*. London: Jessica Kingsley Publishers.

Hogan, S. (2014) *The Introductory Guide to Art Therapy: Experiential Teaching and Learning for Students and Practitioners*. London: Routledge.

Hogan, S. (2015) *Art Therapy Theories: A Critical Introduction*. London: Routledge.

Holtom, R. (1978) Catalogue. In: *The Inner Eye*. Elliot, D. (Ed.). Oxford: Museum of Modern Art. pp. 35–41.

Junge, M.B. (2010) *Modern History of Art Therapy in the United States*. Springfield: Charles C Thomas.

Kaczynski, T. (2020) *Who Am I?: The Story of a London Art Studio for Asylum Seekers and Refugees*. Cheltenham: The History Press.

Kaimal, G., Mensinger, J.L., Drass, J.M. and Dieterich-Hartwell, R.M. (2017) Art therapist-facilitated open studio versus coloring: Differences in outcomes of affect, stress, creative agency, and self-efficacy. *Canadian Art Therapy Association Journal*. 30:2. pp. 56–68.

Kalmanowitz, D. and Lloyd, B. (1997) *The Portable Studio: Art Therapy and Political Conflict: Initiatives in Former Yugoslavia and South Africa*. Great Britain: Health Education Authority.

Kalmanowitz, D. and Lloyd, B. (2005) *Art Therapy and Political Violence: With Art Without Illusion*. London, New York: Routledge.

Kapitan, L. (2008) "Not art therapy": Revisiting the therapeutic studio in the narrative of the profession. *Art Therapy*. 25:1. pp. 2–3.

Killick, K. (2000) The art room as container in analytical art psychotherapy with patients in psychotic states. In: Gilroy, A. and McNeilly, G. (eds.) *The Changing Shape of Art Therapy*. London: Jessica Kingsley. pp. 99–114.

Lloyd, B. and Usiskin, M. (2020) Reimagining an emergency space: Practice innovation within a frontline art therapy project on the France-UK border at Calais. *International Journal of Art Therapy*. 25:3. pp. 132–142.

Luzzatto, P. (1997) Short-term art therapy on the acute psychiatric ward: The open session as a psychodynamic development of the studio-based approach. *Inscape*. 2:1. pp. 2–10.

Lyddiatt, E.M. (1971) *Spontaneous Painting and Modelling: A Practical Approach in Therapy*. London: Constable.

Mahony, J. (2011) Artefacts related to an art psychotherapy group: The therapist's art practice as research. In: Gilroy, A. (ed.) *Art Therapy Research into Practice*. London: Peter Lang. pp. 231–250.

Malchiodi, C.A. (1995) Studio approaches to art therapy. *Art Therapy*. 12:3. pp. 154–156.

Malis, D. (2017) Crafting the visual voice: Art as agency in studio art therapy. *ATOL: Art Therapy OnLine*. 8:1. https://journals.gold.ac.uk/index.php/atol/article/view/438/pdf.

Marshall-Tierney, A. (2014) Making art with and without patients in acute settings. *International Journal of Art Therapy*. 19:3. pp. 96–106.

Martyn, J. (2019) Can exhibiting art works from therapy be considered a therapeutic process? *ATOL: Art Therapy OnLine*. 10:1. https://journals.gold.ac.uk/index.php/atol/article/view/548/pdf.

McGraw, M. (1995) The art studio: A studio-based art therapy program. *Art Therapy*. 12:3. pp. 167–174.

McNiff, S. (1995) Keeping the studio. *Art Therapy*. 12:3. pp. 179–183.

Miller, S.M. (2020) Disability art: Potential intersections in studio practice with artists labeled/with intellectual and developmental disabilities. *Art Therapy*. 37:2. pp. 93–96.

Moon, C.H. (2002) *Studio Art Therapy: Cultivating the Artist Identity in the Art Therapist*. London, New York: Jessica Kingsley.

Moon, C.H. (2016) Open studio approach to art therapy. In: Gussak, D. and Rosal, M. (eds.) *The Wiley Handbook of Art Therapy*. Hoboken: Wiley Blackwell.

Moon, C.H. and Shuman, V. (2013) The community art studio: Creating a space of solidarity and inclusion. In: Howie, P., Prasad, S. and Kristel, J. (eds.) *Using Art Therapy with Diverse Populations: Crossing Cultures and Abilities*. Philadelphia, PA: Jessica Kingsley. pp. 194–200.

Morris, F.J. and Willis-Rauch, M. (2014) Join the art club: Exploring social empowerment in art therapy. *Art Therapy*. 31:1. pp. 28–36.

Nolan, E. (2019) Opening art therapy thresholds: Mechanisms that influence change in the community art therapy studio. *Art Therapy*. 36:2. pp. 77–85.

Nowell-Hall, P. (1978) Catalogue. In: Elliot, D. (ed.) *The Inner Eye*. Oxford: Museum of Modern Art. pp. 35–41.

Omand, H. (2022) Protested space: Artworks made in a therapeutic art studio under threat from cuts. In: Skaife, S. and Martyn, J. (eds.) *Group Art Psychotherapy in the Hostile Environment of Austerity Britain*. London: Routledge.

Potash, J.S., Mann, S.M., Martinez, J.C., Roach, A.B. and Wallace, N.M. (2016) Spectrum of art therapy practice: Systematic literature review of *Art Therapy*, 1983–2014. *Art Therapy*. 33:3. pp. 119–127.

Saotome, J. (1998) Long-stay art therapy groups. In: Skaife, S. and Huet, V. (eds.) *Art Psychotherapy Groups: Between Pictures and Words*. East Sussex: Routledge. pp. 156–180.

Schaverien, J. (1991) *The Revealing Image*. London: Routledge.

Skaife, S. and Huet, V. (1998) Dissonance and harmony. Theoretical issues in art psychotherapy groups. In: Skaife, S. and Huet, V. (eds.) *Art Psychotherapy Groups: Between Pictures and Words*. East Sussex: Routledge. pp. 17–43.

Stepney, S. (2019) Visionary architects of color in art therapy: Georgette Powell, Cliff Joseph, Lucille Venture, and Charles Anderson. *Art Therapy*. 36:3. pp. 115–121.

Thompson, G. (2009) Artistic sensibility in the studio and gallery model: Revisiting process and product. *Art Therapy*. 26:4. pp. 159–166.

Timm-Bottos, J. and Rosemary, C. (2015) Learning in third spaces: Community art studio as storefront university classroom. *American Journal of Community Psychology*. 55:1–2. pp. 102–114.

Vick, R.M. (2016) Community-based disability studios: Being and becoming. In: Gussak, D. and Rosal, M. (eds.) *The Wiley Handbook of Art Therapy*. Chichester: Wiley Blackwell. pp. 829–839.

Walker, C. (1978) Catalogue. In: Elliot, D. (ed.) *The Inner Eye*. Oxford: Museum of Modern Art. pp. 35–41.

Waller, D. (1991) *Becoming a Profession: The History of Art Therapy in Britain, 1940–82.* London: Routledge.

Winnicott, D.W. (1965) *The Maturational Processes and the Facilitating Environment*. London: The Hogarth Press.

Wix, L. (2010) Studios as locations of possibility: Remembering a history. *Art Therapy*. 27:4. pp. 178–183.

Woddis, J. (1993) Art therapy: New problems, new solutions? In: Waller, D. and Gilroy, A. (eds.) *Art Therapy: A Handbook*. Buckingham, PA: Open University Press. pp. 25–48.

Wood, C. (1997) The history of art therapy and psychosis 1938–95. In: Killick, K. and Schaverien, J. (eds.) *Art, Psychotherapy and Psychosis*. East Sussex: Routledge. pp. 219–236.

Wood, C. (2000) The significance of studios. *Inscape*. 5:2. pp. 40–53.

3 How might studios help? Further thoughts on the significance of studios

Chris Wood

A studio is a place to sit and think and a place to make things. It might be a place to be in the company of others or a place for solitude. Studios are physical places – but 'studio' is also a concept that helps me and other art therapists think about the foundations of our practice. Most studios are indoors, but the ideas on which they are based are relevant in outdoor settings. They are significant for service users, hopefully providing a sense of safety, a place to make art, play, and maybe daydream.

Edward Adamson is seen as an art therapy pioneer in the UK. He started working at Netherne Hospital when it housed 2,000 psychiatric patients just after the Second World War. He worked at the hospital for more than thirty years. I have a particular interest in how Adamson was an art therapist because I worked at Netherne in the early 1980s, shortly after he retired. Some of the people I got to know at the hospital had been his patients. They remembered him and spoke to me about his studio work.

One man talked about Adamson's respectful courtesy and the way he would sit down next to him and ask: "Would you like to do some painting?" Another person I met was Rolanda Polonsky. She became well known as an artist. Eventually, she managed to leave the hospital and reclaim something of her life. She spoke affectionately to me of the ways Adamson had responded to her as an artist. Together they had cast her large sculptures; many were put on display in the hospital church. He had not patronised or pathologised her as a long-term patient. In his work with Rolanda and others, it was clear that Adamson's 'studio' work regularly took him outdoors.

Polonsky's sculptures and her drawings give voice to her thoughts about the plight of women. Her take on Christian beliefs put women at their centre. She felt her art making (she made a lot) had been her salvation during the many hard years at Netherne. Her demeanour, especially when making art and speaking about it, turned preconceptions about long-term psychiatric patients diagnosed with 'schizophrenia' upside down. Like many who have strange experiences, she was thoughtful. Also, she was astute in her sense of what others were feeling.

DOI: 10.4324/9781003095606-5

Of his early experiences at Netherne, Adamson writes:

> We were all working very much in the dark in those early days. I must confess that within a few weeks of starting my new job, I was in two minds whether I would have sufficient courage to continue. On looking back I realise that I stayed mainly in response to the overwhelming need of those who queued up every day outside the studio, eager to begin.
>
> (Adamson, 1984: 2)

> I was first offered one of the residents' committee rooms in the hospital for use as a studio. I had discovered some unused rolls of wall lining paper left over from the decoration of a ward, so I cut this up. I had managed to secure some poster paints and brushes. About forty people came to work with me when we first started. They would always be waiting patiently for me outside the door when I arrived to open the makeshift studio.
>
> (Ibid.: 9)

When psychiatric hospitals were home for some 2,000 souls, people were squashed into dormitories with little personal space or dignity. When even the showers were shared, it is not surprising that people queued for their place in Adamson's studio. It was a quiet room (his former patients told me that they were asked to work quietly). It had individual easels and tables arranged in such a way as to provide some personal space (Fig. 6 in Adamson, 1984: 14).

What seems to be our human need for space has been thwarted by political events and by the related struggles we face internally. More than 80 million people in the world are forcibly displaced (Wallis, 2020). Many of these millions have no immediate opportunity for private space and the chance it might give them to know what they think and feel about their lives. They languish in overcrowded refugee camps or attempt to make dangerous crossings at borders. It is hard for the rest of us to imagine what it is to have to stand up and walk away from home, taking only those things we can carry.

Since the international banking crisis of 2008, many governments introduced austerity measures, and without a recovery plan, in the aftermath of the COVID-19 pandemic, these are likely to continue (OECD, 2020). Austerity measures have an impact on the quality of life for the vast majority. For example, few aspects of life in education, employment, health, and the environment have been untouched. In their (2009) book, epidemiologists Wilkinson and Picket use international data sets to show why equality is better for everyone's physical and mental health. In a later book (2018), they consolidate their argument and indicate how income inequality leads to mental distress. Alston's UN report on the UK (2019) uses plain language to show how austerity measures can cause misery. His report compared the Welfare Reform Act of 2012 to the now notorious Poor Law of 1834, which used the dubious distinctions of 'deserving' and 'undeserving poor'. Alston claims such legislation damages physical and mental health; I accept the impact of such legislation on mental health (Wood, 2016b).

In the wake of all these societal issues, how might studios help? The contemporary context could understandably lead to the conclusion that the creation of studios is a minor issue. Nevertheless, this chapter asserts their ongoing significance and the importance of sustaining their place in art therapy practice. Since 2001, I have made a case that methods of therapeutic work are strongly influenced by the social and economic conditions of the time. People no longer queue outside studios in hospital settings. Still, it is not difficult to see that their regular attendance in outpatient, community, and even outdoor settings is motivated by similar needs for places where they can give themselves attention and receive it.

Thinking about the history of art therapy practice and how it has influenced the creation of studios

I have understood art therapy as a meeting place. A strong image in my mind is when a person comes into the studio to join an art therapy group. They have just left their council flat where the flat below has started being used to sell drugs and prostitute young women in the last week. The person is visibly agitated and afraid. In the studio, she has a separate seat and a table. She is welcome and able to paint. Studios are not a panacea, but the relationship with the place, the art making, and the people within them seem to aid resilience.

The need for a place of refuge is understood by most. Still, it is not straightforward to articulate the value of creating spaces for therapeutic work and describe how the issues have changed in response to contemporary social and economic pressures. That the approach of psychological therapies tends to be adapted in response to societal trends is not much explored in any professional literature. Occasionally, there is a comment about the capacity within art therapy to adapt. 'What art therapists seem to do well is adapt to the needs of specific individuals and groups . . . to create safe enough spaces in challenging circumstances and offer flexible approaches to reduce the barriers' (Perry, 2009: 8).

I have written about four historical periods in the development of the UK Art Therapy profession. It is possible to identify three twenty-year periods of the twentieth century and twenty years of the twenty-first century (e.g. Wood, 1997, 2001–1, 2011). Adaptations of therapeutic approaches in these periods echo societal conditions. I briefly indicate where these periods appear in the profession's history before describing how this history has influenced studio use. It is helpful to keep in mind that relevant practitioner publications are often published later than the practice they describe.

In the first period (approximately 1940–1960), art therapists like Edward Adamson and Adrian Hill looked to the power of expression. Studios were usually in hospitals. In the second period (1960–1980), UK art therapists worked alongside other health service workers using ideas from both antipsychiatry and social psychiatry (e.g. Robin Holtom and others writing in Elliot in 1978, and E. M. Lyddiatt described in Thompson, 1989). Studios were still in hospitals but seen

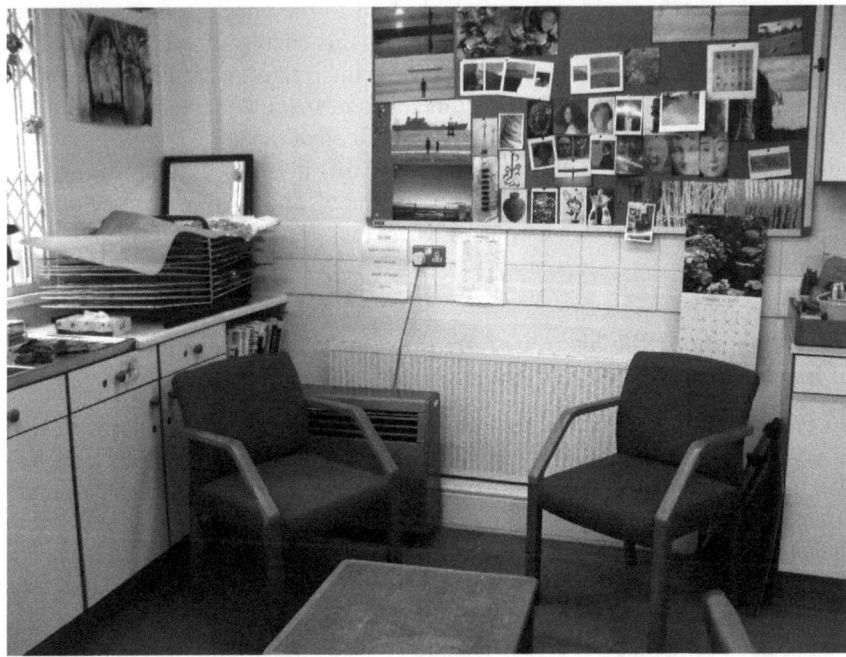

Figure 3.1 A place to sit under the Argyll House studio notice board in Sheffield. The photograph is by Laura Richardson in the NHS Art Therapy studio she created.

as a refuge from the ravages of traditional medical-model psychiatry. (The idea of an escape from psychiatry was not seen as an issue during the first period.) In the third period (1980–2000), there was a push towards community practice, though cuts in public services meant that community work was more impoverished than hoped (e.g. Greenwood and Layton, 1987, 1988). Some hospital studios were lost, and community studios were located wherever space could be found. Many studios were not salubrious, but they continued to provide places for reverie. In the contemporary fourth period (2000–2020 and ongoing), various studios are reported, ranging from purpose-built to improvised sites for art therapy meetings (e.g. Lloyd and Usiskin, 2020; Perry, 2009).

In my publications dated 1985, 1997, 2000–1, and 2014, I grappled with how as art therapists, we create meeting places for work with clients. Success creating studios seems to be helped if we manage to understand what is happening in local settings because of detrimental pressure on services. In writing about the four periods in art therapy, I repeatedly point to how art therapists have adapted. Changes in art therapy thinking about studios are examples of such adaptation (Wood, 2011, 2014).

The economic difficulties provoked by the second OPEC oil crisis in 1979 led to cuts in public sector provision. The OPEC crisis followed the end of the first period of art therapy (described by Adamson in 1984): 'In hospital, people who were denied the luxury of the analyst's couch, nevertheless benefited from reviewing the painful experiences of their past through painting' (1984: 23).

Edward Adamson created and used various studios. One studio was for several people to work in; it had an atmosphere of quiet order. Other studios were for individual artists (e.g. famously William Kurelek, though not all the artists with individual studios were famous). These smaller personal studios were in rooms off hospital corridors and round summer houses dotted throughout the hospital grounds. But as already mentioned, some of Adamson's work was not in studios but outdoors while casting large pieces of sculpture alongside people like Polonsky.

In 1985, I wrote about my fascination with the work of Franco and Franca Basaglia in Italy, and the movement for democratic psychiatry (known as *Psychiatrica Democratica* or PD). In 1978, after a time of global change, the Basaglias and the PD movement managed to get Law 180 passed in Italy. It closed all separate psychiatric hospitals. Their understanding of what was happening to people locked up in terrible run-down psychiatric hospitals, together with a sense of a need for change in Italian society, helped them push for reform. Law 180, against all predictions, has remained on the Italian statute. Law 180 meant that some of the old hospital buildings were transformed into community centres that included studios.

The PD movement made playful, ironic use of the mythological story of the Trojan horse. In the original Greek myth, a giant hollow horse sculpture on wheels was pushed into Troy's walled city, and its hollowed-out innards concealed the invading army. PD also created a horse sculpture. It was built in part of the old Trieste Hospital turned into an experimental art studio. The horse known as Marco Cavallo was made with papier mâché painted blue and placed on wheels. The construction was large, and the battle to get it out of the building became legendary. It symbolised using art in the struggle to get former patients out of hospitals into the community.

In 1997, when I researched the approaches used by art therapists in working with people with a psychosis-related diagnosis, I visited some art therapists to learn how they had created their studios (Wood, 2000–1). The creation and history of studios are rarely described as single subjects but seen in other aspects of the work.

E.M. Lyddiatt's studios provided abundant materials spread over several muddled rooms through which patients could wander and be welcome. She and Robin Holtom worked during the same period of global upheaval on which the Basaglias had based their reforms. Holtom may have been the person who introduced the phrase, 'asylum within an asylum' (in Elliot, 1978) to describe art therapy studios in psychiatric hospitals. This phrase was linked to the criticisms of psychiatry levelled by followers of R.D. Laing. Holtom's studio was in a large disused ward. It had the fertile atmosphere of a garage workshop spilling into a yard. It was a place apart within Springfield Psychiatric Hospital.

As economic conditions in the public sector became harsh in Thatcher's Britain in the 1980s, several prominent art therapy practitioners retreated to private practice. They sought additional training in different analytic and psychodynamic approaches. For the art therapy profession, this influenced the prevailing theory and practice of the time. Until that time, the art therapy profession inclined to be with people in their studios in an ordinary way as possible. Then came a time when more was done to gain psychotherapeutic understanding.

When in 2000–2001, I wrote 'The significance of studios', I grappled with what changes in the times and the approach meant. There was more effort to use art therapy psychotherapeutically. I explained this to myself as the need to gain knowledge as art therapists moved into more independent work in the community. Some understanding was certainly gained, but something about the centrality of art was lost during this period. I wrestled with ideas about traditional art therapy studios (for open studio work) and cooler studios more suited to individual psychotherapeutic work. At this distance, I am not convinced it is possible to make distinctions between just two forms of studio work and in the twenty years since there have been many creative adaptations of practice by art therapists.

I acknowledged that cuts in public-sector finances and the closing of the old asylums meant that some venerable art therapy studios were lost. I did not think that this meant that studios were a lost cause. Instead, I made a case for how studios contribute to service users 'rediscovering' their imaginations. Art therapists come to their practice with rich histories and knowledge of the art world. The studios they create reflect their experience of what has helped them make art. Some might be a place for internalisation and others a simple refuge. Before writing the 2001 paper, I had visited studios created by the art therapist Chris Lyle and her colleagues in Coventry. She memorably said to me that when she first shows a prospective client one of the studios, it is as though she is saying to them: "Here you can feel".

The talk 'From the couch to the council estate: Art Therapy as meeting place' (Wood, 2016a) considered the changing histories of art therapy approaches. It looked at some of the creative ways art therapists had, and continue to, adapt their approach to fit in with local settings and the availability or not of rooms in which to meet. The title is a tongue-in-cheek way of describing the history of approaches.

Having space for mental health work is not a panacea, but physical space and the opportunity for mental space it provides are fundamental. In 2000–2001 (p. 40), what I wrote about our basic need for periods of absorption and about our absorption in whatever we are doing being the opposite of alienation and depression is still relevant. It seems particularly appropriate to an account of studio work in art therapy.

A brief review of themes I find in art therapy literature about studios

Maybe it helps to see the many studio changes during an art therapist's life as part of skilled adaptations. In counting up how many studios I have worked in during my time as an art therapist, I find that there have been ten studios. Some I moved on from as I changed jobs, and for two, I lost the argument. International art therapy literature shows that discussion about studios and their use in different countries spans eight decades. It is not possible to review all of this literature here. Still, the sheer amount of writing implies that studios remain significant, as are the skills of adaptation needed by art therapists in finding a home for their work.

In the UK, there is a parallel history of art therapy studios to that in the US. In 2003, the UK art therapist Nick Moore wrote a passionate review supporting the book by the US art therapist Cathy Hyland-Moon *Studio Art Therapy: Cultivating the Artist Identity in the Art Therapist* (2002). Moore praised the book strongly because he considered that the centrality of art making in art therapy was a contested issue in the UK at that time. In 2010, Wix argues that art making had lost its centrality in US art therapy because of therapists' desire to respond psychologically.

There are understandable concerns in this debate. Some are about the desire for the profession to be taken seriously in skill and practice. Still, a paper by Wadeson (2002) points to the damage inherent in extreme polarisation between approaches in art therapy, those that espouse studio-based practice and the artist identity of the therapist, and those that seek psychological insight. Wadeson tendered the enthusiasm of recently qualified students in her US programme, finding that in 200 final dissertations, they *adapted* to meet the complexity in service-user lives in ways that cannot be reduced to a polarised argument.

Few texts favour studio-based practice exclusively. Nevertheless, most offer thoughtful accounts of the significance of studios in the context of our complicated lives, and most contain a strong implication of the need to adapt.

In her powerful editorial, Kapitan (2008) discusses the collective use of community studios and how they inform practice included in the professional methods of art therapy. She describes how 'ideas on the margins enter into the mainstream and infuse it with new sensibilities that help shape and redefine the field as a whole' (Kapitan, 2008: 2).

A paper on the place of open studios for veterans (Delucia, 2016) offers moving examples showing that studios and linked gallery space provide a sense of belonging and community when returning home feels 'loaded' (p 4). Studios in Delucia's paper offer a transitional stepping stone.

A paper about working with Bosnian refugees in Australia (Fitzpatrick, 2002) includes the word 'home' in its title, and the art therapist works in her client's home. Fitzpatrick points to the value on that occasion of the kitchen table as the studio because it enabled participation by a relative. An understanding of cultural norms was gained that would not have happened in separated individual work.

Kalmanowitz proposes a model that she names 'Inhabited Studio', which offers short group work for people who have experienced war crimes. 'The Inhabited Studio implies the importance of symbolically being able to inhabit' (2016: 76–77) and to find ways of being with difficult emotions. Similarly, Kaimal and Ray's small research study (2017) pointed to how an open studio might enable people to have more of a sense of agency in their ability to work with painful feelings.

The 2010–2012 studio project in the UK saw David Edwards encouraging art therapists to document their studio work experiences. Edwards described the contrast of moving into a purpose-built studio after being alternately frozen and then melted in an abandoned greenhouse:

> This studio smelled of art-making, and more specifically of instant coffee, tobacco, fixative, damp clay, white spirit and paper. While the smell of the room was more or less a constant, it sounded different every day. Sometimes we played music, sometimes we talked or argued or shared a joke, and sometimes we just got on with whatever we were busy doing. It felt comfortable and informal, but at the same time safe and containing. At one time, the majority of art therapists worked in similar spaces to this. Over time, however, such spaces have become increasingly rare.
>
> (Edwards, 2010: 4)

Maybe what can be described as rare is the purpose-built nature of that large Wakefield studio, but the studio as a concept which helps arts therapists practice is not so rare. Edwards curated accounts of the studios written by the art therapists Barrie Damarell, Debbie Michaels, Jo Garber, and Nick Stein in 2011 and Susan Allaker in 2012. That these art therapists had real agency in designing the 'sets' (like stage-sets) for their therapeutic work is evident. They all indicate the containment facilitated by the studios they created.

Similarly, Frances Prokofiev managed to establish a large studio for art therapy work with children in a primary school (Prokofiev, 1998: 44–68). She describes the room as containing many of the materials seen in adult art therapy studios plus toys. Prokofiev offers a thoughtful consideration of the group dynamics and the adaptations necessary to fit into a school context. She sees the room or 'studio' as one of the enabling factors in the work.

Liisa Girard published an account in Finland in 1992 of a project she and colleagues described as 'Adam's Hut'. An illustrated paper about the project was published in English in 2016. Working with a small group of male patients from an acute psychiatric ward, she and her psychiatric colleagues used a hospital outhouse to provide the men with the opportunity to build a shelter. The men concerned had known few actual shelters, and some had been homeless. Girard discusses how symbolically, the building of a shelter helped them (Girard, 2016). The possibilities for collaborating in creating 'shelter' seems to be at the heart of what art therapists hope to provide in creating studios. The gentle work by Girard and colleagues alongside the men and the collaborative art making has contemporary relevance.

A similarly collaborative approach is described in the papers by Greenwood and Layton (1987, 1988). Their description of the 'studio' they used in a community setting humorously foretells something of what was to come in converting multipurpose rooms into temporary but regularly used studios. These papers and those by Girard adopt approaches in-between what I have described earlier as the second and third art therapy periods.

From the turn of this century, there have been many inspiring adaptations to studio use in a fourth period of art therapy history. These have variously used actual studios, the client's home, and work done outside. All offer the opportunity to make art in the context of relationship. However, conventions are changing and developing, as seen in the following three examples from different art therapists.

Jacky Mahony describes a shift in studio practice in which the art therapist makes artwork alongside group clients. 'This practice implies more equality in the relationship between therapist and group members and their interchanges than is usual' (Mahony, 2011: 167).

Julie Harper worked with terminally ill children in their homes, and she shows how a sense of containment in the absence of a studio *may be* preserved within the artwork.

> A young man . . . returned to a piece of artwork he had created two years before . . . it was with great difficulty that he softened the fearsome features and added a pair of wings, completing it two days before his death.
>
> (Harper, 2011: 95)

Rupert Cracknell asks people to use local materials. In Eire, peat was often brought to his studios; it is similar to clay from 'accumulations over aeons: reflecting a fundamental relationship between humanity and the earth and the locations and peculiar features of the places where people live' (Cracknell, 2011: 169).

David Maclagan (2011) challenges an over 'clinification' (see Allen, 1992) of art therapy. He thought the profession neglected its art making core in the push to adopt a psychodynamic approach:

> I shall argue that art therapy is not just a therapy with imagination, but a therapy of imagination: in other words, that before we can depend upon it, imagination itself has to be restored and renewed, not only in the patients we work with but in ourselves as artist therapists.
>
> (Maclagan, 2005: 23)

In addition to Lyle's invitation into a studio with "Here you can feel", Maclagan might show a studio room with the invitation, "Here you can imagine".

Throughout the literature from different periods of art therapy history, I caught glimpses of how skilled art therapists have been in adapting studio work to both services and the socio-economic history of their time. Themes in their writing about studios show how art therapists use studios and a sense of place to help people manage their distress and find their imaginations.

Extraordinary adjustments have been used creatively. Rogers (2002) adapted and made good studio use of an old mortuary. Fenner (2019) found a way of gaining a historical vantage point for understanding the myriad ways the profession has understood the healing potential of having space.

Conclusion: the potential of studios to make a public health contribution

In several papers dated from 2010, 2014 and 2016, I discuss the interconnected nature of human health. I acknowledge this may involve ongoing negotiations for rooms or advocating to use 'Art Therapy as First Aid' (van Laar, 2020) or as an emergency response for migrants (Lloyd and Usiskin, 2020).

It has been fascinating and helpful to discover a discussion of Martha Muchow's study on the life-space of urban children of low socio-economic status living in Hamburg between the two World Wars (Joerchel, 2015). In her research, she indicates how physical space interacts with our sense of identity and psychology. Muchow examined how these children knew the urban places they inhabited and seemed able to move backwards and forwards between intimate, shared, and public space. Joerchel opens the discussion of Muchow's work powerfully: 'Creating a space in which we live, which we enliven, and which enlivens us is a fundamental part of what it means to be a human being' (2015: 546).

The dynamic at the heart of a public health strategy is a need to acknowledge this backwards and forwards movement between the intimate and the public in the lives of the people it serves. Though smaller in scope, this dynamic is also at the heart of the way art therapists use and create studios (Wood, 2014). Art therapists are adaptive and creative in making environments for their work, but they could do more to articulate how their work links to public health politics. Timm-Bottos makes this point well 'too often, I believe, art therapy and other depth psychologies unnecessarily cut the inner warp of psychic work from the outer weave of political life' (2011: 20).

When diagnosed with cancer, the writer, gardener and designer Maggie Keswick Jenks found herself waiting with her husband in a windowless corridor without comfort. Instinctively, Jenks knew that healthcare needs beautiful spaces. Until the end of her life, she worked, creating an inspirational legacy of beautiful places for free holistic cancer-care. There are now some twenty-four stunning buildings in the UK, with a growing network abroad. Photographs of 'Maggie's Centres' online (Medina, 2014) are inspiring, and they show how much is possible. These images give visual support to research on healing environments (Nardo et al., 2010). They might also inspire and support our quest for studios.

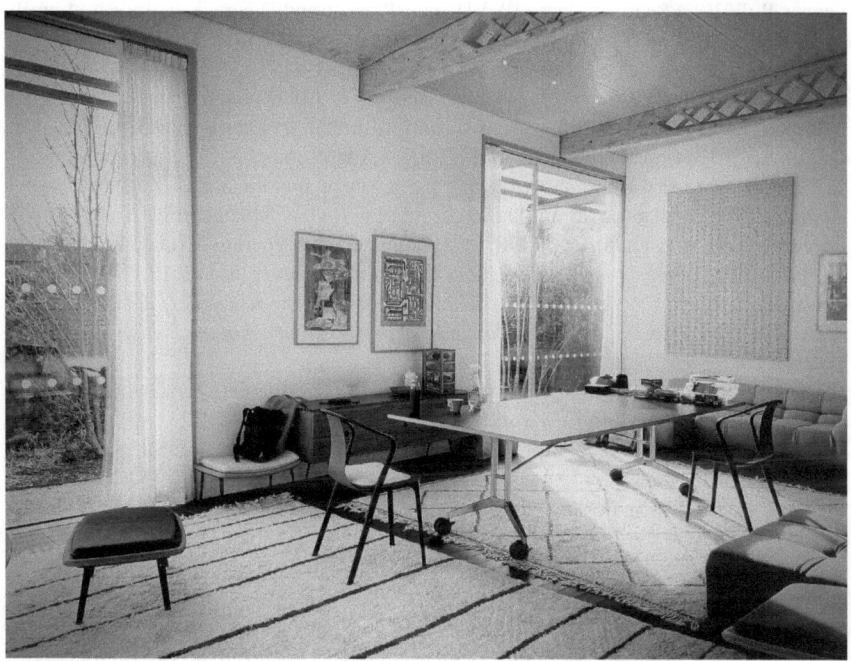

Figure 3.2 Maggie's Centre in Manchester is built with much glass in the middle of lots of plants. It is possible to see its full beauty online. This photograph is by Sangita Mistry of the room at the centre she uses for art therapy.

References

Adamson, E. (1984) *Art as Healing*. London: Coventure.

Allaker, S. (2012) A Piece by Susan Allaker in David Edwards (ed.) Art Therapy Studio Project, *ATOL: Art Therapy Online*, 3:1. Available at: https://journals.gold.ac.uk/index.php/atol/article/view/303/334.

Allen, P. B. (1992) Artist-in-Residence: An Alternative to "Clinification" for Art Therapists, *Art Therapy*, 9:1, pp. 22–29.

Alston, P. (2018–2019) Statement on Visit to the United Kingdom, *United Nations Special Rapporteur on Extreme Poverty and Human Rights*.

Cracknell, P. (2011) Peat. In: Wood, C. (ed.) *Navigating Art Therapy: A Therapist's Companion*. London and New York: Routledge: pp. 169.

DeLucia, J. M. (2016) Art Therapy Services to Support Veterans. Transition to Civilian Life: The Studio and the Gallery, *Art Therapy*, 33:1, pp. 4–12.

Edwards, D. (2010) Art Therapy Studio Project, *ATOL: Art Therapy Online*, 1:1. Available at: http://journals.gold.ac.uk/index.php/atol/article/view/213/228.

Edwards, D. (2011) ATOL Art Therapy Studio Project: A (Re)introduction – David Edwards, Including Pieces from Barrie Damarell, Debbie Michaels, Jo Garber, and Nick Stein, *ATOL: Art Therapy Online*, 2:2. Available at: http://journals.gold.ac.uk/index.php/atol/article/view/293/456.

Elliott, D. (ed.) (1978) *The Inner Eye*. Oxford: Museum of Modern Art Catalogue.

Fenner, P. (2019) A Sense of Place in Art Therapy Practice and Theory. In: Gilroy, A., Linnell, S., McKenna, T. and Westwood, J. (eds.) *Art Therapy in Australia: Taking a Postcolonial Aesthetic Turn*. Leiden and Boston: Brill Sense. pp. 383–418.

Fitzpatrick, F. (2002) A Search for Home: The Role of Art Therapy in Understanding the Experiences of Bosnian Refugees in Western Australia, *Art Therapy*, 19:4, pp. 151–158.

Girard, L. (2016) Construction of Adam's Hut: An Adaptation of Art Therapy for Men Living in the Special Ward of an Acute Psychiatric Hospital in Finland, *ATOL: Art Therapy OnLine*, 7:1. Available at: http://journals.gold.ac.uk/index.php/atol/article/view/403/pdf.

Greenwood, H. and Layton, G. (1987) An Outpatient Art Therapy Group, *Inscape: The Journal of the British Association of Art Therapists*, Summer, pp. 12–19.

Greenwood, H. and Layton, G. (1988) Taking the Piss, *British Journal of Clinical & Social Psychiatry, 6:3, pp. 74–84, Reprinted in Inscape: The Journal of the British Association of Art Therapists*, Winter 1991, pp. 7–14.

Harper, J. (2011) Gentle Dragon. In: Wood, C. (ed.) *Navigating Art Therapy: A Therapist's Companion*. London and New York: Routledge. p. 95.

Holtom, R. (1978) Catalogue. In: Elliott, D. (ed.) *The Inner Eye*. Oxford: Museum of Modern Art. pp. 35–41.

Joerchel, A. C. (2015) Personal Life Space: Learning from Martha Muchow's Classic Study, *Culture & Psychology*, 21:4, pp. 546–565.

Kaimal, G. and Ray, K. (2017) Free Art-Making in an Art Therapy Open Studio: Changes in Affect and Self-Efficacy, *Arts & Health*, 9:2, pp. 154–166.

Kalmanowitz, D. (2016) Inhabited Studio: Art Therapy and Mindfulness, Resilience, Adversity and Refugees, *International Journal of Art Therapy*, 21:2, pp. 75–84.

Kapitan, L. (2008) "Not Art Therapy": Revisiting the Therapeutic Studio in the Narrative of the Profession, *Art Therapy*, 25:1, pp. 2–3.

Lloyd, B. and Usiskin, M. (2020) Re-Imagining an Emergency Space: Practice Innovation Within a Frontline Art Therapy Project on the France-UK Border at Calais, *International Journal of Art Therapy*, 25:3, pp. 132–142.

Maclagan, D. (2005) Re-Imagining Art Therapy, *International Journal of Art Therapy*, 10:1, pp. 23–30.

Maclagan, D. (2011) *Psychological Aesthetics: Painting, Feeling and Making Sense*. London and Philadelphia: Jessica Kingsley.

Mahony, J. (2011) Participative Art Practice. In: Wood, C. (ed.) *Navigating Art Therapy: A Therapist's Companion*. London and New York: Routledge. p. 167.

Medina, S. (2014) The Story of Maggie's Centres: How 17 Architects Came to Tackle Cancer Care, *Arch Daily*, 27 April. Available at: www.archdaily.com/498519/the-story-of-maggie-s-centres-how-17-architects-came-to-tackle-cancer-care accessed 29 August 2020. ISSN 0719–8884.

Moon, C.H. (2002) *Studio Art Therapy: Cultivating the Artist Identity in the Art Therapist*. London: Jessica Kingsley.

Moore, N. (2003) Review of 'Studio Art Therapy: Cultivating the Artist Identity in the Art Therapist, *Inscape: The Journal of the British Association of Art Therapists*. 8: 2, pp. 80–82.

Nardo, D. F., Saulle, R. and Torre, G. L. (2010) Green Areas and Health Outcomes: A Systematic Review of the Scientific Literature, *Italian Journal of Public Health*, 8:7, 4, pp. 402–413.

Organisation for Economic Cooperation and Development. (2020) *Global Economy Faces a Tightrope to Recovery*, June. Available at: www.oecd.org/newsroom/global-economy-faces-a-tightrope-walk-to-recovery.htm accessed August 2020.

Perry, N. (2009) *Reach Out, Outreach: Community Art Therapy for Children and Adolescents*. Unpublished MA Dissertation: Leeds Beckett University.

Prokofiev, F. (1998) Adapting the Art Therapy Group for Children. In: S. Skaife and V. Huet (eds.) *Art Psychotherapy Groups: Between Pictures and Words*. London and New York: Routledge. pp. 44–68.

Rogers, M. (2002) Absent Figures: A Personal Reflection on the Value of Art Therapists' Own Art Making, *Inscape: The Journal of the British Association of art Therapists*, 7:2, pp. 59–71.

Thompson, M. (1989) *On Art and Therapy*. London: Virago.

Timm-Bottos, J. (2011) Endangered Threads: Socially Committed Community Art Action, *Art Therapy*, 28:2, pp. 57–63.

van Laar, C. (2020) *Art Therapy First Aid – Experiential Video Workshop*. Available at: https://carlavanlaar.com/art-therapy-first-aid/ accessed June 2020.

Wadeson, H. (2002) Confronting Polarisation in Art Therapy, *Art Therapy*, 19:2, pp. 77–84.

Wallis, E. (2020) UNHCR: Numbers of Displaced People in World Passes 80 Million, www.infomigrants.net/ accessed March 2020.

Wilkinson, R. and Picket, K. (2009) *The Spirit Level: Why Equality is Better for Everyone*. Great Britain: Allen Lane.

Wilkinson, R. and Picket, K. (2018) *The Inner Level: How More Equal Societies Reduce Stress, Restore Sanity, and Improve Everyone's Well-being*. Great Britain: Allen Lane.

Wix, L. (2010) Studios as Locations of Possibility: Remembering a History, *Art Therapy*, 27:4, pp. 178–183.

Wood, C. (1985) Psychiatrica Democratica and the Problem of Translation, *Inscape: The Journal of the British Association of art Therapists*, Late Issue 1, pp. 9–16.

Wood, C. (1997) The History of Art Therapy and Psychosis (1938–95). In: Killick, K. and Schaverien, J. (eds.) *Art, Psychotherapy and Psychosis*. London: Routledge. pp. 144–171.

Wood, C. (2000–1) The Significance of Studios, *Inscape: The Journal of the British Association of Art Therapists*, 5:2, pp. 40–53.

Wood, C. (2001) *Art, Psychotherapy and Psychosis: The Nature and the Politics of Art Therapy*. PhD Thesis: The University of Sheffield Library.

Wood, C. (2010) Convivencia: A Medieval Idea with Contemporary Relevance, *ATOL: Art Therapy Online*, 1:1. Available at: http://journals.gold.ac.uk/index.php/atol/article/view/218/233.

Wood, C. (2011) Introduction. *Navigating Art Therapy: A Therapist's Companion*. London and New York: Taylor Francis Group: i–xii.

Wood, C. (2014) Private and Public Spaces of Hope in Architecture and Therapy, *ATOL: Art Therapy OnLine*, 5:2. Available at: https://doi.org/10.25602/GOLD.atol.v5i2.367.

Wood, C. (2016a) From the Couch to the Council Estate: Art Therapy as Meeting Place. Keynote Lecture for Finding Spaces, Making Places: Exploring social and Cultural Space in Contemporary Art Therapy Practice, Art Therapy Conference 2016: Goldsmiths, University of London.

Wood, C. (2016b) Back from the Margins: Strange Experiences and Art Therapy, *ATOL: Art Therapy OnLine*, 7:1. Available at: https://doi.org/10.25602/GOLD.atol.v7i1.404.

4 The influential idea of the studio in the thinking and practice of US art therapists

Lynn Kapitan

Introduction

My entry into the conversation about the role of the studio in art therapy began more than twenty years ago with a painting of a dream I'd had while I was researching the loss of creative vitality among art therapists in the US (Kapitan, 2004). In my dream a heavy metal door had slammed shut, leaving just a tiny sliver of blue peeking from beneath its threshold. I longed for that blue to have much more space, so I painted the dream image reimagined as an invisible door opening into clear blue sky. As a space of freedom that is protected yet constrained, I saw the art therapist's studio as a threshold between moving forward with agency in the world and stepping back to rest and reflect upon it. The studio, as I have always understood it, opens the door to renewal and reinvention.

At the time of my dream image US art therapists were coping with a rapidly changing healthcare system that was having dramatic effects on practice. Over the years, art therapy had expanded from traditional psychiatric settings to a diverse breadth of treatment in schools, shelters, outpatient and community mental health agencies, medical hospitals, family therapy settings, group homes, detention centres, and more. But as the US healthcare system grew and diversified, public funding shifted to private insurers, compelling art therapists to adapt to much briefer services, much larger caseloads, and constant pressure to be recognised in the measurable outcomes and pragmatic language of the clinic. Enormous energy was required to keep up with licensing and certification, mandated curricula for graduate training, and longer, more expensive master's degrees in a market that often did not reward them with higher salaries or promising positions. As a result, many art therapists were feeling depleted, discouraged, and disenchanted with our profession.

In 1992, Pat Allen published a paper that became a rallying cry against what she called the 'clinification' of art therapists, referring to a process of subsuming our artistic identity in order to prove ourselves to the clinical establishment. Although Allen based her claim primarily on her own story of ambivalence with her clinical training and its psychodynamic roots, her essay resonated among US art therapists. A rebellion against clinification entered the conversation and initiated a re-centring of the studio in many US art therapists' ideas and conception of practice.

DOI: 10.4324/9781003095606-6

I will attempt in this chapter to capture this compelling spirit of the studio in the theories and practices of art therapists in the US, based on a close reading of the literature and my own perspective. More than a physical space or set of principles and practices, I will argue that, for US art therapists, the studio occupies a deep place of knowing that beckons them 'home' whenever they feel a need to revitalise themselves or reconfigure their profession in a constantly changing world.

The studio in historical narratives

Looking back, I have wondered why clinification, coined by Allen nearly thirty years ago, became such a definitive marker in the discourse on studio approaches to art therapy in the US that still reverberates today (see for example, Fish, 2019; Franklin, 2021; Potash et al., 2016; Timm-Bottos, 2016). The juxtaposition of the studio as a desired alternative to traditional art therapy seems rooted in the tensions of an earlier era, between two major orientations long promoted in the US: Edith Kramer's 'art as therapy' approach, with its focus on the healing capacity of the creative process, and Margaret Naumberg's 'art psychotherapy' in which art making is adjunctive to therapeutic change (Junge, 1994). This dichotomous conception of art therapy accompanied the founding of the American Art Therapy Association (AATA) in 1969 and contentious early debates on how art therapy was defined and practiced. Because these ideas were documented in the prominent voices of Association founders, many pioneering art therapists – who preceded or were unrecognised by the founders or had learnt their craft from unnamed, influential sources – were left out of the historical narrative. They formed an untold story of art therapy's 'aesthetic, art-centered past' in which making art was central (Wix, 2010: 178).

When Wix researched the history of art therapy and marvelled how it had been narrowed to a 'U.S. east coast psychological phenomenon' (2010: 181), she was thinking of the country's geographic heartland where the roots of the art therapy studio are found in the early- to mid-twentieth century work of the artist Mary Huntoon and the enduring, humanistic influence of the Menninger Clinic in Kansas. In 1934, Huntoon created a studio-based therapeutic milieu for Menninger patients that included a vibrant art studio, gallery of patient art, and museum project comprising more than 3,500 works. According to Wix's (2000) archival study, Huntoon contended that the clinic's studio was a place of treatment, not diagnosis; 'therapy is in 'the process' and in the patient's seeing his ideas expressed' (as cited in Wix, 2000: 171). Grounding her theories on aesthetic rather than psychiatric tenets (calling diagnostic interpretation of art 'malarkey'), she contended that the creative process and its therapeutic power must be allowed to establish itself within a studio atmosphere. Like her British contemporary Edward Adamson, Huntoon considered the art therapist's role as a catalyst in this process.

The US Midwest produced several early proponents of studio-based art therapy, a number of whom can be traced back to the Menninger Clinic. Two founders of the AATA, Don Jones and Robert Ault, were fine artists who worked at Menninger, beginning in 1951 and 1960, respectively. Charles Anderson, a visionary

Black art therapist, was hired by Ault in 1962 and spent his long and distinguished career there (Stepney, 2019). Jones later moved to Ohio to establish an art therapy programme in a psychiatric hospital where Bruce and Cathy Moon, two contemporary US art therapists associated with the studio approach, were trained and mentored. Ohio was also home to an enduring studio art therapy programme created by Mickey McGraw in 1967 in collaboration with a medical centre (McGraw, 1995). At Chicago's School of the Art Institute, Don Seiden taught sculpture while practicing at a major hospital before founding the school's art therapy degree programme. In reference to the dominant narrative of the time, a bemused Seiden recalled hearing 'what was happening on the East Coast' that trickled 'back to him in the midlands [about] something called art therapy' (Vick, 1996: 193).

But geography is not the only location in the narrative of art therapy's studio past. Prominent among those who insisted from early on that art therapy was larger than the binary of art and psychotherapy were pioneering US art therapists of colour (Potash et al., 2016). Georgette Powell practiced in New York City in the 1930s during the Harlem Renaissance, a major visual arts movement of African American artists. Her artistic vision of art therapy was rooted in community activist work as a master artist at Harlem Hospital (Boston and Short, 2006). Cliff Joseph, who was present at the formation of AATA, aligned his art therapy practice with social protest artists of the US civil rights movement and the impact of the Black experience on his own art and the art of racially and economically diverse populations (Stepney, 2019). These and other voices like Lucile Venture, Wayne Ramirez, and Sara McGee established art therapy in social action and diverse cultural traditions; they understood that to be accessible to socially marginalised communities, a broader, less limiting framework was required (Doby-Copeland, 2019; Potash et al., 2016).

Knowing the full history of art therapy locally and abroad is important because our beliefs are formed and constituted by the narratives we tell and retell. Historical figures in a profession's folklore often become fixed into archetypes – to be emulated or to be rebelled against, their deeds and words embodying professional identity. Other voices and perspectives are lost. Consequently, in the US, the studio has often been positioned on one side of an artificial divide that is not reflected in actual practice (Potash et al., 2016). When understood as a hybrid with diverse, multidisciplinary roots, however, art therapy can begin to appreciate its art-based legacy as a constantly renewable source of connectivity and potential (Wix, 2010).

Rhizomatic roots in the narrative of the studio

The studio in US art therapy can be understood in the context of movement across a continent, and across time, space, and culture. Forty times the physical size of the UK, the US is home to over forty graduate-level degree programmes in art therapy. Art therapists train in art schools and medical colleges, research universities, and small liberal arts colleges. Their education in art therapy reflects not just regional differences in artistic and psychological orientations but the mingling and cross-pollination of ideas from the first to second, third, and even fourth generations of art therapists, resulting in a breadth and plurality of theories and practices. With each generation, a new, more diverse cohort of art therapists infuses the framework with new configurations of knowledge. This focus on ideas rather than dominant history allows for exploration and connection between early concepts to current outcomes.

Because of its breadth and diversity, we might think of art therapy in the US as not solely a profession but a social geography of interconnected habitats, where communities of practice share a common purpose and knowledge base of practices, resources, and perspectives (Kapitan, 2014; Wenger, 1998). How we inhabit art therapy depends upon our standpoint or position in this landscape, our trajectories through it, and our ways of aligning and realigning with it over time. Thus, whenever we discuss the theories and practices of the field, and the place of the studio within them, what we are actually doing is presenting different parts of the landscape to each other and persuading others of their importance (Kapitan, 2014).

The influential idea of the studio in this configuration can be understood as an orienting means by which art therapists find interconnections – between *here* and *there, then* and *now* – that help them revise their working theories in response to new problems and thinking within the place-relatedness of their practices. In the studio we might pick up a chalky pastel, say, and make a swish of colour across the paper that draws our attention to an old sensation or surprising feeling surfacing anew, bearing witness to the current reality we find ourselves in. Following the phenomena that arise in art making, we may welcome or interrupt their arrival and, in the process of forming new expressions, become more attuned to our context and needs. Because these and further connections can reproduce and join with others in any direction from any spot, the studio fosters a *rhizome* (Deleuze & Guattari, 1980/1987) or underground network of thoughts, ideas, and theories, which on the macro level link art therapy communities of practices into a single, highly complex system.

In the imagination of US art therapists, the rhizome has also been observed by Timm-Bottos (2016) as appearing in liminal spaces of psychic innovation and by Wix, who saw art therapy studios as 'places of possibility where diverse ideas and disciplines intersect' (2010: 181), through relationships with other makers, materials, and artworks. McNiff, a prominent voice in the discourse, has long observed the studio's 'creative ecology of forces' that simultaneously grow from and act upon people and their artworks (1995: 179).

When I investigated the phenomena of disenchantment among US art therapists (Kapitan, 2004), what came forward in their stories, again and again, was a feeling of being cut off from a source they knew their therapeutic practice depended upon. They longed for reconnection in the studio, described metaphorically as a personal or communal taproot into a great underground river. Art making drew up vital waters of a reciprocating creativity; when they lost connection with this primal source, they felt they'd lost a crucial, nourishing part of themselves. In contrast, those who had incorporated studio practice into their work could tolerate or neutralise more disturbance in their environments and appeared to be more resilient to toxic stress. When I revisit their stories from my perspective of today, I recognise the signs of hidden rhizomatic roots that, if nurtured, can regenerate when broken. Perhaps, this is the trust in the process (McNiff, 1995) that art therapists call forth to ground themselves. Connectivity in the studio provides a pathway through parched lands to the vital waterholes that replenish and make people whole again.

The rhizomatic narrative of the studio understands the deep longing for rest and 'at home-ness' in all this movement of time and space, as well as the persistent warning of clinification that has come to mean neglect of an art therapist's core identity. As to the latter, however, two clarifications are needed. First, art therapy in the US exists in a far more complex landscape than it can or should be reduced to an oppositional dichotomy of studio versus clinic. With its rhizome-like capability, engagement in any practice that generates creative vitality invites wholeness, frees up life-affirming energy, and returns the individual to the sympathies, resonances, and empathies that connect people.

Second, the resonance felt by the notion of clinification may be less about fear of or resistance to assimilation into the clinical world than a reclaiming of the studio as a source of creative vitality that houses the heart's longing. Wix suggested that the resurgence of studios in the US discourse highlights a hunger for heartfelt learning, about 'what is loved and longed for in art therapy studio practices and maybe even the larger field itself' (2010: 182). Others perceive the studio as linked to a desire for personal freedom and a persistent, encouraging yearning for somewhere else (Heywood, 2009) – for a different kind of life, a different way of being with oneself or with others, or a different relationship with the world.

Orienting concepts and reclaimed contexts

It is somewhat ironic for me to be writing about the studio, considering that I've never had the privilege to design such a space. The first studio spaces I ever worked in were borrowed classrooms, lunchrooms, utility closets, and even my car. Later, as I leaned into this fate, I brought art therapy into community spaces – plazas, shelters, church patios, board rooms, open fields, and back porches. My practice was affirmed by Kalmanowitz and Lloyd's (1999) concept of the *portable studio* as not a room or physical site but an art therapist's internal frame of reference that has allowed me to hold and adapt to whatever spaces I find myself in. This dynamic 'studio' must be acutely alert to the context and its cultural values, social and political dynamics, potentiality, and vulnerabilities within a complex web of relationships (Kalmanowitz & Lloyd, 1999). Reyhani Ghadim (2020) conceives of the art therapist as not simply a catalyst but a *nomadic force*, moving into spaces and across systems and territories while being guided by a creative flow that grounds the work in imagination, strength, and personal or collective power.

Nothing in this description suggests a rejection or absence of therapeutic or even clinical skills; it resists polarities. Rather, the construct of the studio serves a proliferating expanse of professional practices that characterise art therapy in the

US today. Among many examples is Nolan's (2019) community art therapy studio that expands access to care by offering a nontherapeutic pathway into therapy for some participants and a supportive pathway out of therapy for others. The studio-gallery model developed by DeLucia (2016) with war veterans reclaims the public space of art exhibition for rituals of community-wide healing and dialogue. Drass's community studio within a medical model setting deploys the ethos of punk rock to create a 'culture of connection' (2016: 138) that builds resiliency. We have yet to learn the results of art therapy's paradigm shift to virtual studio practice in the global pandemic, but US studio frameworks appear sufficiently flexible to meet essential therapeutic needs.

New conceptual language for describing art therapy as a contemporary art practice is emerging in the US discourse, with antecedents in Robbins's (1993/2000) notion of *therapeutic artistry* that draws out the artist in both the therapist and patient to move the therapeutic process along. Thompson's (2009) concept of an *artistic sensibility* towards life's challenges extends this idea. Stereotyped identities that have been pathologised as 'other' and apart from a healthy society break down in the studio and recentre on an artist's self-agency. Awareness of an 'artistic self' permits a perceptual freedom and responsiveness to internal processes and the external environment, which serves clinical treatment and other forms of practice. Moon (2016) described such responsiveness as central to *relational aesthetics* on which art therapy practice is grounded.

Contemporary practice revises the triadic relationship of art, therapist, and client (Schaverien, 1992) by reclaiming and incorporating the wider, surrounding context as another relational partner. Hospitable, collaborative help is invited in, whether from the physical space or from cultural guidance, history and political structures, extended family members, benign spirits, and ancestors. When everything in therapy is perceived within a practice of artistry, patterns of connection across all such influences frame relational-artistic practice (Moon, 2016). 'This thinking and acting gives me a sense of agency within oppressive contexts', Moon wrote. 'I am not a victim of circumstances but an artist subtly disrupting habits of power and privilege, challenging them in small, subversive ways' (2016: 60). Beyond clinical intervention, art therapy has evolved into a powerful social practice (Kapitan, 2014).

We now have language to understand art therapy's hybridisation differently as well. The field has long straddled art and therapy, but they need not be static, bipolar positions. The trap of a bipolar framework is that it offers only two terms to be juxtaposed or combined, whereas true hybridisation allows for an endless number of associations and permutations (Vigneron, 2011). Art therapy in the US today is an ecosystem that, when flexible and sensitive enough, can shift boundaries to accommodate new needs. From the studio we have learnt that the places where we meet, cross boundaries, and build new relationships are particularly potent. Known in the biological world as *ecotones*, these overlapping habitats – where 'our kind' meets 'your kind' – always produce tension but also diversity and complex exchange dynamics from which a whole new kind of hybrid may evolve (Kapitan, 2015).

The nature of an ecotone may explain some of the tensions that accompany art therapy throughout the world wherever it has attempted to put down roots. The idea may begin with a juxtaposition of pre-existing elements that overlap, oscillate, or jockey for position. This dynamic tension produces a course correction at times, and sometimes factions that split off from the field's unifying rhizomatic roots. Gradually, a true hybrid arises that becomes rooted in and perceived as organic to its context shaping over time (Vigneron, 2011). The studio in US art therapy has had this trajectory, as a creative force that is always unravelling supposedly settled ideas of art therapy's place, identity, and origins.

Conclusion

In the current era of globalisation and rapid change, historical struggles to establish art therapy may appear, with hindsight, to have been insufficiently fluid, open, and dynamic; centred more on defining art therapy's boundaries than the diverse contexts that surround and shape it. But it is very hard to root in a constantly shifting world. In the studio we tap into a primal source, asking not only 'who are we?' but also and more insistently, 'how can we be 'at home' in movement?' The studio in US art therapy is a vital incubator for new ideas and practices that will infuse creative vitality and knowledge of art therapy far into the future. There we balance on a threshold between what we are and our becoming of something else.

References

Allen, P. (1992) 'Artist in residency: An alternative to "clinification" for art therapists', *Art Therapy. Journal of the American Art Therapy Association*, vol. 9, no. 3, pp. 22–28, https://doi.org/10.1080/07421656.1992.10758933.

Boston, C. & Short, G. (2006) 'Notes: Georgette Seabrook Powell', *Art Therapy: Journal of the American Art Therapy Association*, vol. 23, no. 2, pp. 89–90, https://doi.org/10.1080/07421656.2006.10129649.

Deleuze, G. & Guattari, F. (1987) *A thousand plateaus, capitalism and schizophrenia* (B. Massumi, Trans.). University of Minnesota Press, Minneapolis. (Original work published 1980).

DeLucia, J.M. (2016) 'Art therapy services to support veterans' transition to civilian life: The studio and the gallery', *Art Therapy: Journal of the American Art Therapy Association*, vol. 33, no. (1), pp. 4–12, https://doi.org/10.1080/07421656.2016.1127113.

Doby-Copeland, C. (2019) 'Intersections of traditional healing and art therapy: Legacy of Sarah McGee', *Art Therapy: Journal of the American Art Therapy Association*, vol. 36, no. (3), pp. 157–161, https://doi.org/10.1080/07421656.2019.1649548.

Drass, J.M. (2016) 'Creating a culture of connection: A postmodern punk rock approach to art therapy', *Art Therapy: Journal of the American Art Therapy Association*, vol. 33, no. 3, pp. 138–143, https://doi.org/10.1080/07421656.2016.1199244.

Fish, B.J. (2019) 'Response art in art therapy: Historical and contemporary overview', *Art Therapy: Journal of the American Art Therapy Association*, vol. 36, no. 3, pp. 122–132, https://doi.org/10.1080/07421656.2019.1648915.

Franklin, M. (2021) 'Expanding artistic literacy in art therapy education: Self-reflection tools for assessing artwork and art-based research', *Art Therapy: Journal of the American Art Therapy Association*, vol. 38, no. 1, pp. 22–32, https://doi.org/10.1080/074216 56.2020.1721993.

Heywood, I. (2009) 'Making and the teaching studio', *Journal of Visual Arts Practice*, vol. 8, no. 3, pp. 195–204, https://doi.org/10.1386/jvap.8.3.195/1.

Junge, M. (with Asawa, P.) (1994) *A history of art therapy in the United States*, American Art Therapy Association, Mundelein, IL.

Kalmanowitz, D. & Lloyd, B. (1999) 'Fragments of art at work: Art therapy in the former Yugoslavia', *The Arts in Psychotherapy*, vol. 26, no. 1, pp. 15–25, https://doi.org/10.1016/S0197-4556(98)00027-6.

Kapitan, L. (2004) 'Artist disenchantment and the collaborative witness project', *Journal of Pluralism, Pedagogy, and Practice*, vol. 3, no. 1, art. 7, https://digitalcommons.lesley.edu/jppp/vol3/iss1/7.

Kapitan, L. (2014) 'Re: Invention and realignments of art therapy', *ATOL: Art Therapy OnLine*, vol. 5, no. 1, https://journals.gold.ac.uk/index.php/atol/article/view/328/359.

Kapitan, L. (2015) 'Arts therapies in the ecotone: Contact, collaboration, and creative entanglement', Keynote Address presented at the Joint Conference of the Australian and New Zealand Arts Therapy Association and the Australian Creative Arts Therapy Association, Adelaide, Australia, 18 October.

McGraw, M.K. (1995) 'The art studio: A studio-based art therapy program', *Art Therapy: Journal of the American Art Therapy Association*, vol. 12, no. 3, pp. 179–183, https://doi.org.10.1080/07421656.1995.10759154

McNiff, S. (1995) 'Keeping the studio', *Art Therapy: Journal of the American Art Therapy Association*, vol. 12, no. 3, pp. 167–174, http://doi.org/10.1080/07421656.1995.10759156.

Moon, C.H. (2016) 'Relational aesthetics and art therapy', in J. Rubin (ed.), *Approaches to art therapy*, 3rd edn, Routledge, New York.

Nolan, E. (2019) 'Opening art therapy thresholds: Mechanisms that influence change in the community art therapy studio,' *Art Therapy: Journal of the American Art Therapy Association*, vol. 36, no. 2, pp. 77–85, https://doi.org/10.1080/07421656.2019.1618177.

Potash, J.S., Mann, S.M., Martinez, J.C., Roach, A.B. & Wallace, N.M. (2016) 'Spectrum of art therapy practice: Systematic literature review of *art therapy*, 1983–2014', *Art Therapy: Journal of the American Art Therapy Association*, vol. 33, no. 3, pp. 119–127, http://dx.doi.org/10.1080/07421656.2016.1199242.

Reyhani Ghadim, M. (2020) 'Nomadic art therapy: A contemporary epistemology for reconstructed practice', *Art Therapy: Journal of the American Art Therapy Association*, https://doi.org/10.1080/07421656.2020.1746617.

Robbins, A. (2000) *The artist as therapist*, Jessica Kingsley, London. Original work published in 1993.

Schaverien, J. (1992) *The revealing image: Analytical art psychotherapy in theory and practice*, Routledge, New York.

Stepney, S.A. (2019) 'Visionary architects of color in art therapy: Georgette Powell, Cliff Joseph, Lucille Venture, and Charles Anderson', *Art Therapy: Journal of the American Art Therapy Association*, vol. 36, no. 3, pp. 115–121, http://doi.10.1080/07421656.2019.1649545.

Thompson, G. (2009) 'Artistic sensibility in the studio and gallery model: Revisiting process and product', *Art Therapy: Journal of the American Art Therapy Association*, vol. 26, no. 4, pp. 159–166, https://doi.org/10.1080/07421656.2009.10129609.

Timm-Bottos, J. (2016) 'Beyond counseling and psychotherapy there is a field. I'll meet you there', *Art Therapy: Journal of the American Art Therapy Association*, vol. 33, no. 3, pp. 160–162, https://doi.org/10.1080/07421656.2016.1199248.

Vick, R.M. (1996) 'An interview with Don Seiden', *Art Therapy: Journal of the American Art Therapy Association*, vol. 13, no. 2, pp. 191–197, http://doi.org/10.1080/07421656. 1996.10759219.

Vigneron, F. (2011) 'Hybridization in the visual arts: Now you see me, now you don't', *Visual Anthropology*, vol. 24, pp. 30–45, https://doi.org/10.1080/08949468.2011.525457.

Wenger, E. (1998) *Communities of practice: Learning, meaning, and identity*, Cambridge University Press, Cambridge.

Wix, L. (2000) 'Looking for what's lost: The artistic roots of art therapy: Mary Huntoon', *Art Therapy: Journal of the American Art Therapy Association*, vol. 17, no. 3, pp. 168–176, https://doi.org/10.1080/07421656.2000.10129699.

Wix, L. (2010) 'Studios as locations of possibility: Remembering a history', *Art Therapy: Journal of the American Art Therapy Association*, vol. 27, no. 4, pp. 178–183, http://doi. org/10.1080/07421656.2010.10129388.

5 Studio Upstairs

A working arts studio with a therapeutic concern – beginnings

Claire Manson, Douglas Gill, and David Fried

'All life can be framed within art'.

– Douglas Gill

Introduction

Studio Upstairs opened on 10 October 1988. It was named Studio Upstairs (courtesy of Douglas Gill) as a reference to the studios in people's heads, and that we were at the top of the Diorama Arts building three steps from the roof. Built to house a diorama, a precursor to the cinema, the building had a large octagonal central space where the audience would have been rotated as light from the high glass dome illuminated paintings. It was a massive rabbit warren of seemingly endless rooms. Now the Prince's Trust, it had various incarnations, from Hydrotherapy Centre to Diorama Arts.

Diorama Arts, a legal squat, was an artist's collective of visual artists, musicians, disability arts group, theatre companies, 'Play Space', a photographer, editors, and at one point the Philadelphia Association. In return for keeping the building from total disrepair and paying the rates, the Crown Estate allowed this arts community to thrive. When approached with the idea of opening a studio for people often deemed 'mad', Diorama Arts were interested in a group that straddled the arts and psychotherapy. Although there was reluctance by Diorama Arts for us to hang our first show 'Bats Out of the Belfry' in 1990, by the time of our second, 'Insider, Outsider' in 1992 we were very well supported.

The studio has continued to mount exhibitions on an annual basis at a variety of venues, with people choosing to exhibit or not. This has been an essential component of studio practice, which contrasts with standard art therapeutic practice.

In 2000, at $-20°C$, a group of studio artists with Claire Manson mounted an exhibition at the State Russian Museum's education department, St. Petersburg, travelling a long way from the day hospital or psychiatric ward.

After five years in the Diorama we moved to a nearby ex-industrial building. We lost our semi-circular rooftop studio with a bath in one corner and a hole in

DOI: 10.4324/9781003095606-7

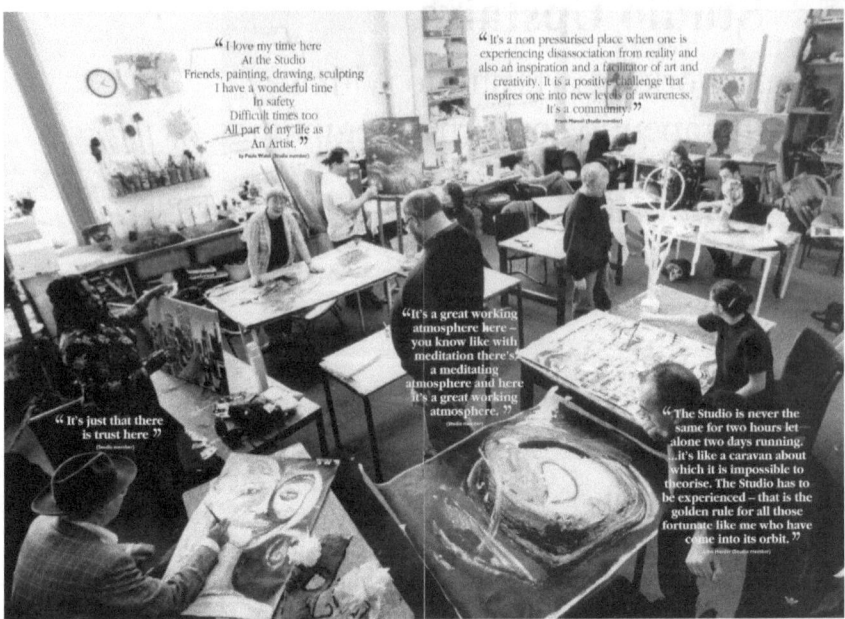

Figure 5.1 The second studio at Diorama Arts. Photograph from Studio Upstairs annual
report 1996/7.

the roof, where magnificent fungi grew, and found ourselves in solid rooms with
central heating. It was a loss, but part of our evolution. Starting with one day a
week, the studio opened an extra day every eighteen months until full-time and,
eventually, from receiving £5.00 a day via social workers who approved it as
a placement for their clients, as more formal contracts came in under Margaret
Thatcher, we were rubber-stamped as an approved provider of 'mental health' services. We had spot contracts with local authorities across London, and to keep our
independence we refused block contracts, earning the accusation of being '*very
1970's*'. Constituted as a registered educational charity and limited company in
1997, in 1999, Douglas Gill moved to Bristol and established the second studio at
Spike Island art centre. In 2006, studio London moved to Hackney, East London.
Under the current valued directorship of Zlatinka Histrova, the third studio was
established in Croydon in 2017.

Studio Upstairs was set in motion by Douglas Gill, Claire Manson, and Jo Bat-
terham (nee Hill), who met when studying art therapy at Goldsmith's College at
the end of the 1970s. David Fried, a co-author of this chapter, trained in fine arts
at the Royal College of Art prior to his art therapy training. He has worked in NHS
psychiatry for thirty years and at Studio Upstairs for over twenty years, keeping
continuity of ethos and approach.

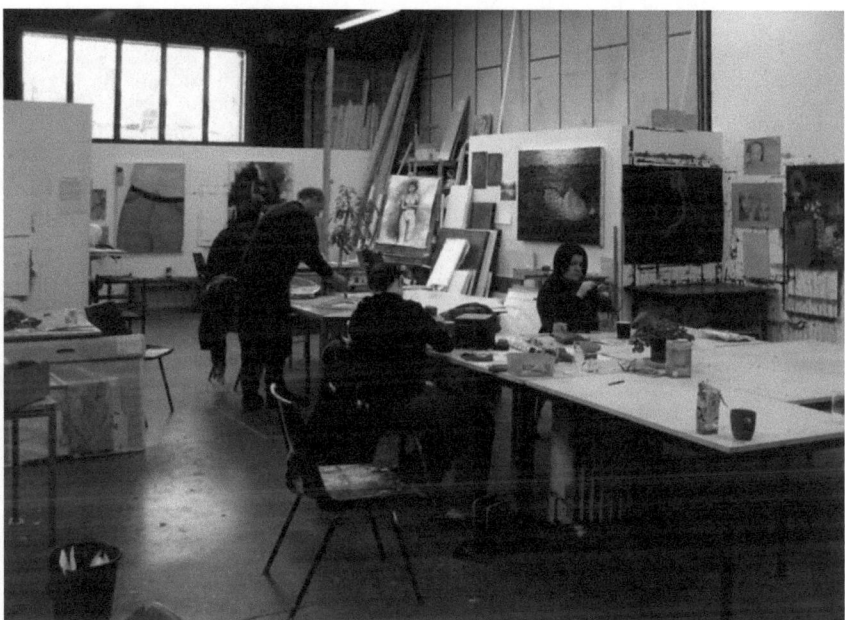

Figure 5.2 Studio Upstairs Bristol. Photograph from Studio Upstairs archive.

Some pre-history that informed the decision to create a studio and its practice

Prior to art therapy, while studying at Dartington College of Arts, Douglas Gill participated in a workshop with the American performance artist Carolee Schneemann, which propelled him into performance art, fringe theatre and the community arts movement. These were extraordinary times where artists from different disciplines were not only collaborating in the production of public works but also overlapping with health and education. After training in art therapy he undertook further training in psychotherapy with the Philadelphia Association, founded by R. D. Laing. It was here, in discussions with his training supervisor, that the seeds were sown to form a community art therapy project in the building.

Claire Manson was a working studio potter. Post Goldsmiths, she worked in psychiatric hospitals running art therapy rooms. Having attended sixteen educational establishments, she was acutely aware of how marginal we can feel (and can become) and of the profound need for true facilitating environments.

Jo Hill, a fine artist, was working as an art therapist in various settings. Through her continued art practice, she knew intrinsically the power and value of art making in a social environment and of exhibiting.

When we started the Studio, we were not aware of anything comparable in the landscape. The three founders were of the opinion that the models of art

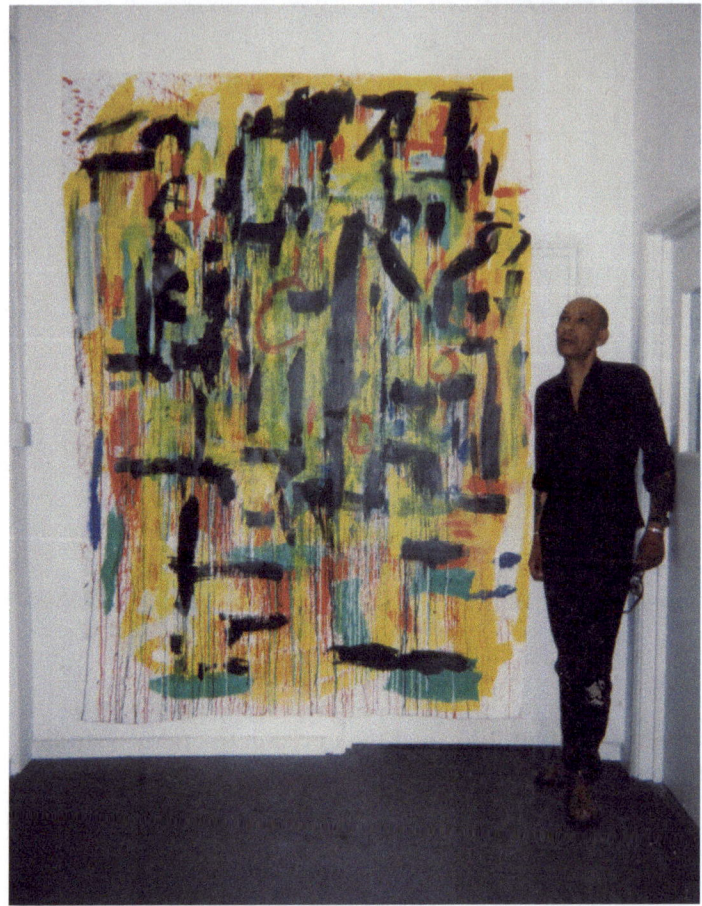

Figure 5.3 Studio Upstairs artist Paul Burke and his work. Photograph from Studio Upstairs archive.

therapy they had been taught during their training had to some degree relegated art making to a subsidiary component of what was essentially a psychoanalytically informed model of psychotherapy, utilising the art image to facilitate communication within the relationship. They wanted to establish an arts studio for people who had a variety of psychological experience, often extreme and traumatic, outside the conventional educational and psychiatric establishments. They wanted to sidestep the clinical or treatment notion of art therapeutic intervention by establishing a studio firmly located within the arts community that would primarily engage in art making of various kinds, with communal, educational, and therapeutic components integrated into the fabric of the ongoing ordinary relationships within the studio environment.

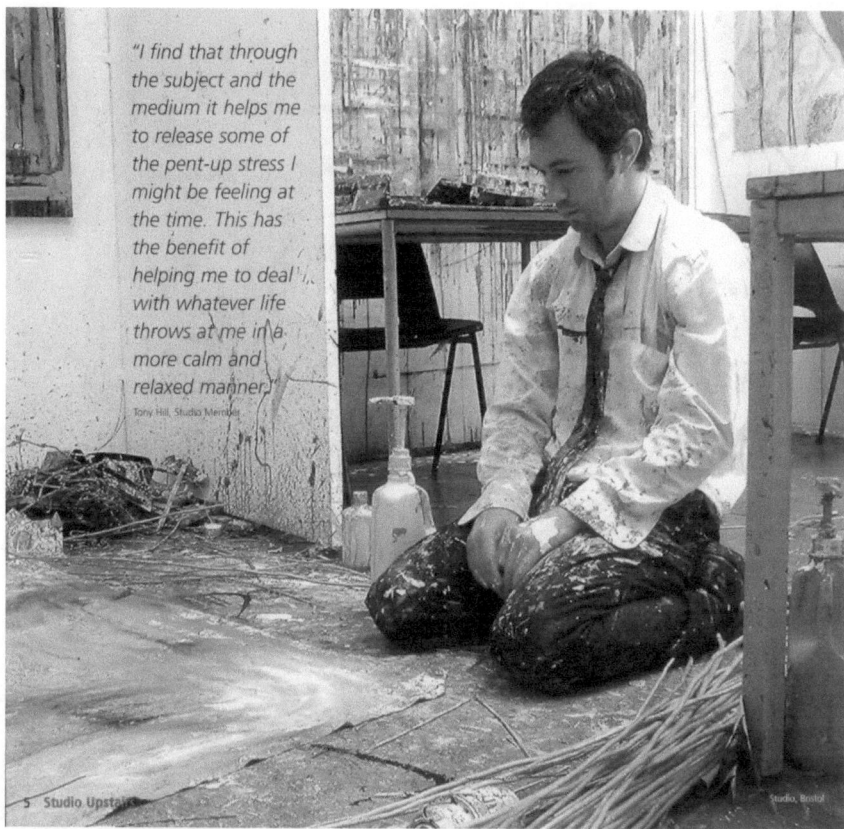

"I find that through the subject and the medium it helps me to release some of the pent-up stress I might be feeling at the time. This has the benefit of helping me to deal with whatever life throws at me in a more calm and relaxed manner."

Tony Hill, Studio Mercian

Figure 5.4 Studio Upstairs artist Andy A'Court painting. Photograph from Studio Upstairs annual report 2003.

The Studio has always been open for a full working day, rather than sessional therapy time. Within this extended time people could come and go as they pleased, but regular commitment was always expected. Gradually, as the studio's reputation grew, more and more people became members. Many people were referred by statutory services while others found their own way to the studio, having heard about it through the grapevine and made an agreed self-funded payment each day. People attending engaged in an experience of art making and communication, utilising their psychological and emotional experiences of life as the raw materials of their creative experimentation.

In other environments, this material might have been sanitised, rationalised, pathologised, or viewed as a symptom of disturbance and dysfunction. At Studio Upstairs people's experiences were, and are, viewed in a phenomenological way as valuable and meaningful. Always interested in the person and their experiences

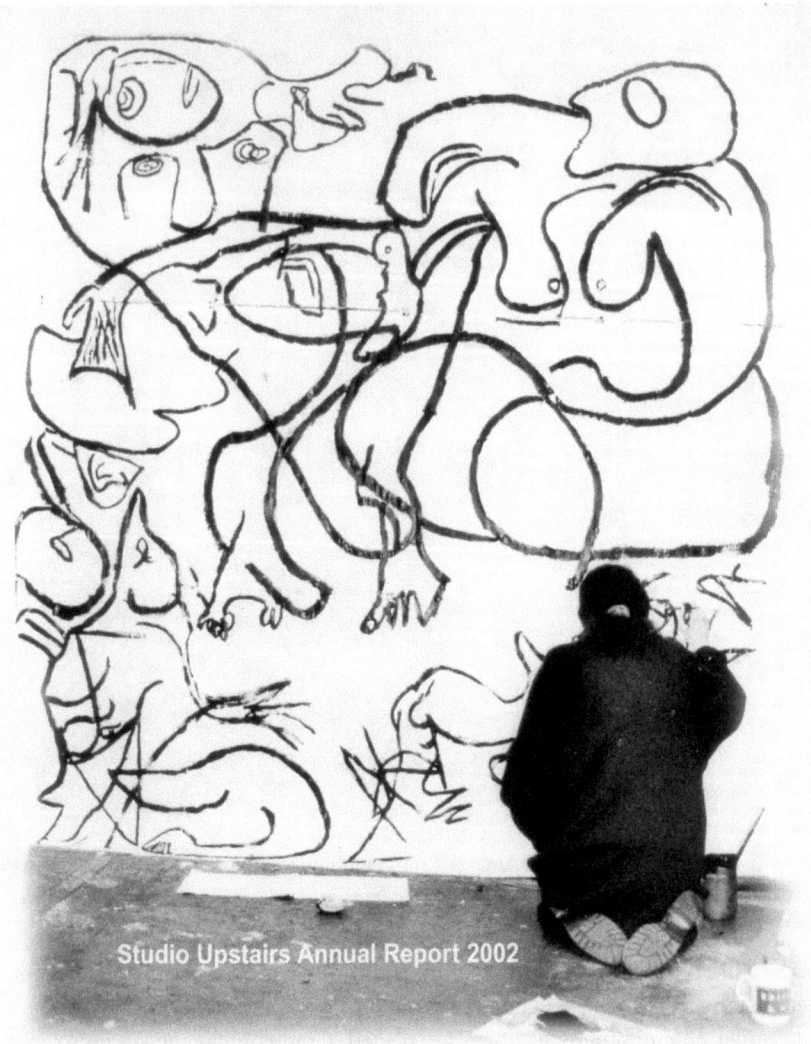

Figure 5.5 Studio Upstairs artist Diane Butler at work on a large-scale painting. Photograph from Studio Upstairs annual report 2002.

but not interested in medicalising, there has simply been a respect for people no
matter what their educational, mental health background or status. Within this
framework of respect for people and their thinking, everyone was invited into participation in an ongoing conversation that was relational and intersubjective rather
than being a treatment procedure. Although an alternative provision we liaise with
the statutory sector when circumstances require.

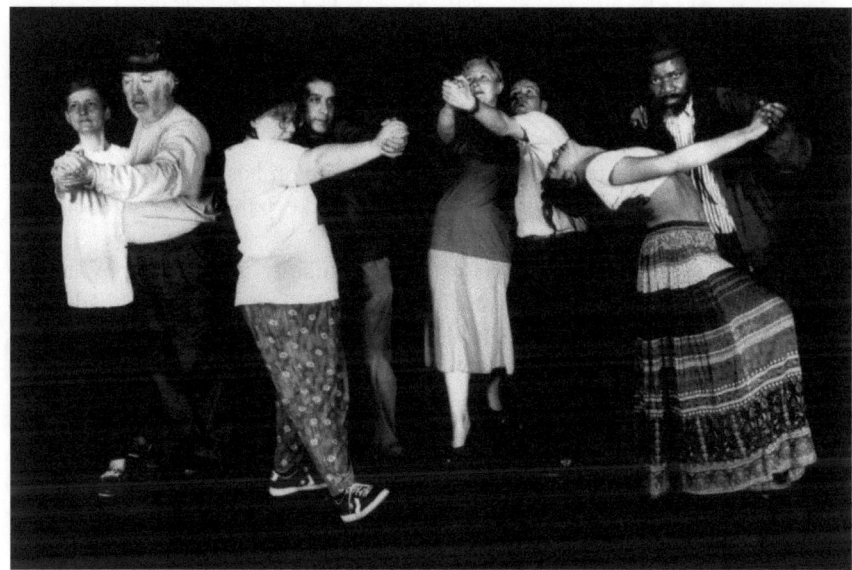

Figure 5.6 The Studio Upstairs performance group. Photograph from Studio Upstairs annual report 1998.

Alongside the visual arts studio, performance, poetry, and music groups were established with the same principles. The idea was to have a diversity of art forms that could fertilise and complement one another. Studio membership became a vital sustaining component in the lives of many. Studio Upstairs sits between health, education, and community – inviting people into a conversation about arts practice, history, education, psychoanalysis, politics, aesthetics, the price of bread – it's all present in the studio. Our intention has been to go beyond the confines of the rational to uncover creative potential, an idea at the heart of surrealism, a movement sometimes seen as a precursor to art therapy, one which was also wary of psychiatric interpretation as echoed in this quote by Salvador Dali:

> *If you understand your painting beforehand you might as well not paint it.*
> *(Dali, 1992: 15)*

Ethos and practice – a conversation with Doug, Claire, and Dave

CLAIRE: Within the philosophical framework we created it was a collaborative venture, welcoming the input of numerous people over the years, disputes and all, including studio managers, students, members, administrators and volunteers. Each one, in their own capacity, influenced and contributed to the evolving ideas and life of the studio.

It was very collaborative, but not all free and interchangeable. Initially, we wanted a flat structure but learnt, very painfully, that we had to have a hierarchy and we learnt much about organisational overview and responsibility, with supervision soon becoming a vital underpinning of the work.

DAVE: Without idealising, the work at Studio Upstairs could be described as a labour of love, because the financial remuneration has been low compared to the commitment and input that is required to keep the studio functioning.

The underlying influences were in part the community arts philosophy and in part the therapeutic communities established by R.D. Laing and the Philadelphia Association. For example, at Kingsley Hall in Bow, East London during the 1960s and early 1970s and by extension, existential phenomenology and post-modern philosophy.

CLAIRE: It was very purposefully a studio in an arts centre and a deliberate side-step away from art therapy – people were not *in treatment*. We worked hard to keep ideas alive by questioning entrenched language that keeps people in their role and were very thoughtful about the language we used. For example, never using the word clinical and using 'studio manager' not therapist, which was perhaps a bit clumsy, but we wanted to try to deconstruct the expectation of the patient/therapist – a very powerful dyad. We wanted to open it up, to keep questioning. As one person asked, "what is a therapist, can I not be a therapist, am I not also able to think about another?" There are no 'service users' at the studio, but members, artists.

We all cheered when at our first exhibition, visitors complained they didn't know who the 'clients' were and some suggested the studio managers, whose artwork was also on show, should wear badges saying who they were.

DOUG: But we did acknowledge that we were art therapists. It was only because we were art therapists that we had the licence to be able to explore another way of looking at the therapeutic value of art. The art therapy profession was overtly disapproving and going into the public gallery was an anathema. I loved the title of the first show 'Bats out of the Belfry'; seventy pieces of work in three galleries and we were all wondering if it was going to be alright and of course people loved it and it was a very successful show. It was flying in the face of the doubts of the profession and many years later when the profession started to talk about art being at the heart of their practice, we thought, well that's actually not always been so. The difficulty with putting on the first show at Diorama Arts was that the artists' community there did not want us putting up 'mad art'. We were so challenged. When we opened, we encountered the same response from the artistic community as we had from the psychiatric and art therapy communities.

Visiting professionals would ask, "Where's the therapy?" and we would say, "it's wall to wall!" It's art in a therapeutic space, as we came to say, eventually. It was not an open studio because it was never closed. It was not a closed art group because it was never a conventional group. It was whoever happened to be there. But it was not a casual drop in either, it was made up of whoever was inhabiting that space and how they were influenced and affecting one another. It was our responsibility along with the students, volunteers, and other people coming into the studio to hold that space and to think about it in different ways. We used to say: it's a very hard job we ask of people coming here to work because, to quote Steve Gans, the philosopher and psychoanalyst the team used to meet with for supervision, "*You have to take the white coat off, that's just a cover story*".

CLAIRE: You have to be there, like in any relationship and a bit more. Think about your presence, because you are holding people who are coming in from quite extreme psychological moments and experiences into a different space. It was about Respect with a capital R, we were always talking about respect. You have got to be yourself so that you can be present as a person and as an artist. We would talk with each other in an open way, and it was not that our roles were confused between being a studio member and a studio manager. We always talked about boundaries; never clear in any relationship.

DOUG: This is why I coined the term 'Therapeutic Arts Community'. It's all there, we're all in it and we're all participating, generating that kind of thinking, we created a culture.

A visiting psychoanalyst asked us, "How can you hold psychosis in an art studio?" How do you hold psychosis in an art studio? Well, in that case what the psychoanalyst does not understand about art is that, in a way, it is already psychotic as the psychosis is already there. It is like asking how can you hold a person in art? People are simply held in art, it's not that we hold them, the art does!

Most of the time it is assumed that speech is a given, but with people who you are unable to speak with, the power of the arts come into play. It is in the nature of psychosis that people are beyond everybody, including themselves, but this does not prevent someone from making marks, making artwork, this is where they are held. We are providing a facility where people can be held even though they may be beyond us to communicate with.

DAVE: When working in a continuous session from 10am to 5pm, one is very exposed. One has to be oneself. It is the only way to maintain an authentic presence. In one way it is easy, but in another way it's hard to do. It's not treatment but an exploration. If we spend some time not necessarily exploring you or exploring me but just exploring, then perhaps we will reach a point where things will begin to untangle or unravel, and things will start to appear before us.

CLAIRE: Yes, it's an exploration and how can you further marginalise people when you are interested in the person and their thinking? It's important that the exploration is never fixed.

DOUG: This has been one of our greatest problems at Studio Upstairs – it was always evolving and never in one place. The exploration was a continuum for the project. It's intersubjective. It's not like one person has the overview or the knowledge. One creates a solid enough frame and within that frame people can explore. The exploration can be unpredictable, that is the nature of art. It is mercurial.

In the studio there was no prohibition, anyone entering it had the opportunity of giving form to any of their experiences. This then is the 'frame of art'. Coming from the arts we are very taken by frames, which seems to me to be at odds with boundaries in therapy. Boundaries are prohibitions creating the image of guards at a perimeter that one cannot go beyond. The frame, on the other hand, is a contained space that also makes reference to what is outside the frame, whereas a boundary will always be at the limit.

DAVE: Within the physical and emotional framework of the studio, you have the space set up. You have the materials and equipment; you have the cups of tea. This continuity makes it possible for people to work because you then have the continuity of the known and predictable and reliable setting that permits the exploration and experimentation.

CLAIRE: It was a working studio, where the art was of primary importance. We took fine art seriously. We have to be able to continue to experiment and begin to be able to experience the difference between an internalised critical voice and the sense of wrong that comes with aesthetic decisions.

CLAIRE: Early on, there was a man who attended the studio who'd been prosecuted for murder; looking cadaverous and somewhat threatening, he easily fell into a stereotype. He was helped in his legal fight by a prominent campaigning journalist and found innocent. When he attended the studio he said, *"This is the only place that I have attended where there is an ongoing discourse about me. I am not chopped up into pieces like an hour of art therapy in a Day Centre"*. It was the continuity, held in the frame of the space, the time, the materials, and the studio community. As we would say:

'We invite people away from the identity of psychiatric patient at the margins of society, into the identity of artist, the artist's community. A valued place.' Douglas Gill.

'Through the making of art, the Studio was a Midwife for people.' Claire Manson

DOUG: Right from the beginning it was very clear how studio practice was indelibly bound up with culture, hence an art centre, and that this was a fundamental move away from health. Being seen in the studio and then in the public gallery generates a high level of anxiety, which it was our task as studio managers to manage and contain.

CLAIRE: In 1995, I talked about 'stage fright' in a paper for a conference in Russia (on arts, health and education). 'The Tolerance of Being Seen – The Unbearableness of Not' wondering about how we step onto the stage, walk through the door – dare we move from '*isolation to relation*?' (*Steve Gans*). We can all be vulnerable in the face of others. As you've noted Doug, 'how frightened we all are of each other'.

DOUG: The mindset of going into a hospital is completely different, it is that of going into a treatment centre, but Studio Upstairs was not that.

CLAIRE: From isolation to community. Perhaps we were a bit idealistic, perhaps we still are?

DOUG: The community arts movement was a very strong thing. It was just about making art ordinary and madness ordinary. Anyone can make a bit of art, a piece of theatre or music or whatever the gig is. Community arts was just as strong an influence as that of Laing and the Philadelphia Association (PA). We were doing the same thing as the PA in terms of their therapeutic households. Established places where people could learn to live together separate from psychiatry.

At the time when Studio Upstairs was emerging, contemporary arts culture was changing hugely. It was familiar for artists to be in analysis. It was no longer just the familiar forms of painting and sculpture. It was okay to go anywhere that you felt it was meaningful to go. I think that spirit was around in the studio in terms of what could happen and what could take place, the freedom of which was encapsulated in our motto '*All Life Can Be Framed Within Art*' (1997). You don't have to dictate what that frame is.

CLAIRE: Studio Upstairs was about the shared sensibility of individuals involved in different capacities. Within our shared sensibility we brought our different experiences and perspectives. These differences kept the discourse and creativity alive; it was the essential nature of the studio. Crafting the studio always felt like making a piece of sculpture.

Many people have been influenced by the studio's approach and its flexibility; hopefully, they have been able to take that with them. Some people have been in the studio for a very short time and some people have been there for years. There was no fixed time scale for attending and this is in complete contrast to the prevalent treatment model of today where everything has to be evidenced and time limited. Sometimes, there is nowhere else to go.

DAVE: The ethos was influenced by the community arts movement along with the ideas of R.D. Laing and the Philadelphia Association of dismantling the hierarchical structure of the psychiatric and therapeutic relationship. For example, the psychiatric patient would often find themselves in a disadvantageous position should they question the authority of the mental health professional or institution's perception and treatment of them. We do not deny that sometimes people need psychiatric treatment, but often the treatment that people receive is stifling and unimaginative and at times it can be a form of oppression, in that it can impose many restrictions and can disregard the value and significance of the patient's experience.

CLAIRE: Through our evolution we wanted people to develop their art, to learn, and not be left helpless in a regressive relationship having to re-enact and feel like a baby, helpless again, which is very powerful and useful within psycho-therapy but not what Studio Upstairs was about. We saw there was a place to teach, I recall David Maclagan talking about aesthetics. Art therapists seemed not to talk about aesthetics as if when you begin to look out at your world and measure and weigh and see the form, was not seen as part of development. We respected 'mad' people (whatever mad means) and knew that people just wanted to be able to learn. People are constantly intellectually marginalised just because they have had or are having extreme psychological experiences, much of them traumatic.

DAVE: We introduced aspects of art school practice. For example, having reviews of peoples' work and having life drawing sessions with naked life models (much frowned upon by various art therapists and social workers!). I have been interested in an aspect, of art education in the studio, which consists of starting a conversation where you can look at the work itself and try to evalu-ate it within a constructive critical framework, rather than allowing people to remain in a state of fusion with their work. It is our view that constructive critical discussion forms part of the studio relationship and work. It is derived from an educational approach but also part of the group and individual thera-peutic process. This has to be handled very carefully because many people can have a fragile ego structure and may find any criticism of their work as being a direct attack; If I am my work and you criticise my work, then you are devaluing me – as can be felt by many students in art and drama education. We prefer to create more of a thinking space between a person and their work as part of an analytical educational therapeutic process.

DOUG: It is not just anything goes either. There is a rigour to it and how you main-tain this rigour. It's all in the development of the culture. It is not acceptable that anything goes but, at the same time, do anything you feel is right and let's see what's going on.

CLAIRE: A lot of people have been sabotaged by education and when people are very delicate, they can often break down when faced with certain challenges. Good education must be about helping people to not feel damned to their core because you damned their work. Good therapy is good education. Bad therapy is educative. We sometimes learn more from our mistakes than we do getting it right. There is no such thing as a mistake in art, how do we find what works without making marks that don't?

DAVE: A central working principle of Studio Upstairs is the sharing of the space. People attending are required to show some consideration towards others; don't be selfish, tidy up after yourself, use materials and equipment responsi-bly. It is all part of being in the community. Building awareness and looking after one another. It's not patronising. It's ongoing, like the washing-up. We want to humanise the encounter at an interpersonal and relational level. In the studio, the encounter is between individuals who have different roles and responsibilities.

We are born naked into the social, but to navigate and negotiate this is a development; hence the power of community and of therapeutic community.

Additionally

Studio managers do their own artwork whilst being practically and emotionally available to the studio members in a variety of ways. Some people want technical, artistic, or educational support; others want emotional and psychological support, or a variety of these elements.

Studio managers manage the space in order to facilitate the creative work of the studio. The main emphasis is on art making, and the therapeutic work is discreet and takes place within the ordinary interpersonal relationships between everyone in the studio. Essentially, we are trying to establish a meeting between human beings with a more equal relationship, encompassing a broader view of the person, their identity, and perspectives. Within this relationship, there are still boundaries that underpin the work and make a containing space in which it is possible for people to develop both their artwork and a capacity to connect and relate.

It is a space where there is belief in, and respect for, the capacity of people diagnosed with a whole range of psychiatric conditions to assume the responsibility of being sane in madness and to be trusted to have the capacity to be functional in dysfunctionality without denying the madness or dysfunctionality.

We attach importance to maintaining a space for despair and negativity to be expressed, communicated, and explored in general through conversation and artwork, in the same way that positivity is allowed to be communicated in equal measure – to make interesting, disturbing, and thought-provoking work. We want to really embrace the various creative forms fully in their own right, in an exploratory capacity, and not as a subsidiary component of an art therapeutic practice: working as artists, allowing time for formulation of an image or an idea for as long as it takes. In this way, the creative act draws deeply on a shared humanity in making art. Jean Dubuffet was an artist who collected psychiatric art and coined the term 'Art Brut'. He says:

> *In the realms of art, genius abounds and any newcomer has sufficient reserve to produce an admirable work of art.*
>
> *(Musgrave and Cardinal, 1979: 1)*

The therapeutic aspect is integrated into the fabric of the normalised studio interaction and communication. The whole community can at different times be therapists for one another even though we have different responsibilities. But we are equal as artists, working alongside one another and allowing ourselves to be influenced by one another.

We consider that it is important, at whatever level, to immerse oneself in the physical and mental process of art making. We want people to become absorbed with the handling and use of different materials in this process, and the studio is committed to developing serious art practice, using good artists materials, good quality paints, and drawing materials.

We are less concerned about knowing the meaning of an image in the process of its creation. We want the freedom for the manifestation of the process to take place without the potential hindrance of the definition or speculation of what something might mean either to the maker or the viewer. The meaning of the image can be speculated about or explored if it becomes relevant or desired.

> *To talk aesthetically, technically, emotionally, or to remain silent if they wish.*
> *Douglas Gill and Claire Manson*

There is meaning to be found by the maker or the viewer. Meaning is there to be explored more in depth as part of the conversation if wished. One is inevitably visible through one's own images and this is an absolutely essential form of participation as the way to be in the studio, whether member or studio manager.

Managers are required to be artistically skilled and knowledgeable as well as being therapeutically skilled and knowledgeable.

Fine arts, and the development of people's creative drive, is fundamental to the Studio. This naturally extends to visiting galleries, museums, and theatres not only providing food for thought but also allowing us to experience being with each other outside the confines of the studio space. The studio has always been about people looking further beyond the doors of the family home or the psychiatric ward.

The studio continues to evolve to meet the demands of the changing economic climate and prevalent treatment philosophy of the statutory sector funders, while still trying to retain the essential working approach that we developed. We are interested in the long-term therapeutic change and artistic growth within the lives of people attending the studio and hope to continue for as long as we can, evolving and expanding this eclectic creative therapeutic approach. During the thirty-two years of its existence innumerable members plus volunteers and art therapists have passed through the studios. Over this time, a large portion of members managed to significantly reduce their reliance on psychiatric services. The studio communities have provided a place where people can work, think, and communicate with one another irrespective of designation.

It's always difficult to know where things begin, and in the making of a piece of artwork, where do we end? We hope to keep many thoughts and questions open, to allow the next thought, the next mark or sound to be made. There is so much more we could say, but here we meet the boundary of the chapter.

References

Dali, S. (1992) *50 Secrets of Magic Craftsmanship*. Dover Publications, London.
Musgrave, V. and Cardinal, R. (1979) *Outsiders: An Art without Precedent or Tradition*. Arts Council, London.
Studio Upstairs. (1997) *Annual Report 1996/7*. Studio Upstairs, London.

Selected bibliography

Buber, M. (1923) *I and Thou*. Scribner Classics, New York.

Cabanne, P. (1971) *Dialogues with Marcel Duchamp*. Thames and Hudson, London.

Cooper, R. (ed.) (1989) *The Philadelphia Association Papers, Between Philosophy and Psychoanalysis*. Free Association Books, London.

Crumb, R. (1967–68) *Zap Comix no's 0 & 1*. Print Mint, San Francisco

Dali, S. (1935) *My Pictorial Struggle*. Julien Levi, New York.

Ehrenzweig, A. (1970) *The Hidden Order of Art*. Paladin, London.

Heidegger, M. (1978) *Basic Writings*, Ed. David Farrell Krell. Routledge, London.

Kierkegaard, S. (1843) *Fear and Trembling*. Penguin Classics, London.

Laing, R. D. (1965) *The Divided Self*. Pelican Books, London.

Laing, R. D. (1971) *Self and Others*. Pelican Books, London.

Merleau-Ponty, M. (1964) *The Primacy of Perception*. Northwestern University Press, Illinois.

Outsiders exhibition. (1979) *Haywood Gallery*, Curators Victor Musgrove, Roger Cardinal, London.

Prinzhorn, H. (1922) *Artistry of the Mentally Ill*. Springer-Verlag, Berlin.

Sartre, J. P. (2000) *Nausea*. Penguin Classics, London.

Storr, A. (1976) *The Dynamics of Creation*. Pelican Books, London.

Szasz, T. (1961) *The Myth of Mental Illness*. Harper & Row, New York.

Thompson, M. (1997) *On Art and Therapy*. Free Association Books, London.

6 Art therapy in an art school

Learning through studio practice

Philippa Brown

Introduction

In this chapter I discuss, through an educational lens, the importance of studio practice for student learning on the art therapy programme at the University of Hertfordshire. Formerly situated in the School of Art in St Albans, the art therapy training, from its inception in the 1970s, developed a strong affinity with the visual arts placing the artistic development of the art therapist central to the knowledge and understanding of therapeutic practice (Waller, 1991). The chapter explores the historic and influential relationship art therapy has with the art school and how studio practice offers the trainee a stronger relationship to artistic practice in the development of becoming an art therapist. When the artwork made by a trainee crosses the boundary from the 'open studio' to either the art school's media workshops or the closed experiential groups, the dynamics at play shift and, along with this, the meaning. This processing and engagement through various settings allows for a nuanced understanding of the service user's experience of art therapy and contexts.

The educational context

In the mid-twentieth century, experiential learning in the visual arts was first seen in Germany at the Bauhaus and subsequently in the US at Black Mountain College. Both institutions formed radical ideas in pedagogy that prioritised the artistic process as a key educational and learning activity. Notably, Black Mountain College took a democratic approach to staff and student collaborations that maintained a vision of the visual and performing arts as interrelated and profoundly life enhancing (TATESHOTS, 2016). After the Second World War, the residue of these progressive approaches flourished in British Art Schools where, in the 1970s, St Albans School of Art established one of the first art therapy trainings in the UK. The art therapy training at St Albans School of Art was founded on a vision of creative synergy between the disciplines of the visual arts, where it is recognised for promoting the artistic development of the art therapist, an ethos that continues to attract students to this day (Waller, 1991; Elkins, 2001).

DOI: 10.4324/9781003095606-8

Art therapy's historical roots with arts education, from the early to mid-twentieth century, are extensively documented by Waller (1991) in her book *Becoming a Profession: The History of Art Therapy in Britain 1940–82*. In the past decade, higher education has been radically changed into a politically and economically driven system dependent on increased student numbers and rising fees (Davis, 2011). Consequently, this transformed educational landscape has significantly impacted on teaching and learning, away from the purity and heritage of experimentation in art making as a primary learning tool, to a more applied approach across all arts disciplines and Health and Care Professions Council (HCPC) approved courses.

Art therapy at St Albans School of Art

Waller (1991: 236) makes it clear that in the 1970s, the path to securing a national professional training in art therapy, between the British Association of Art Therapists (BAAT) and St Albans School of Art, were fraught with acrimonious debate. Despite the disharmony, the school principal Antony Harris recognised the value of art as a therapeutic discipline and a potential educational cooperation within the School of Art. In pursuit of this academic quest, Harris brought Edward Adamson on board and together they created a Certificate in Remedial Art. Adamson provided a legacy of being both an arts educator and art therapist, a dialectical relationship acknowledged by Harris in the St Albans School of Art archive (2020) when he says 'the therapeutic value of art education cannot be ignored . . . The importance of visual arts in remedial situations cannot be questioned'. Harris and his successor John Evans, another pivotal figure at the School, worked towards educational recognition and professional status for art therapy through academic rigor. As academics, they argued for a melding in the curriculum of the disciplines of fine art, visual perception, psychology, psychiatry, and social sciences, an expansive body of knowledge they knew would underpin the application of art therapy at local health and welfare services (Waller, 1991).

In 1977, when I undertook the Postgraduate Diploma in Art Therapy, Edward Adamson taught on the course, where he held a weekly 'open studio' to support our art practice. I was strongly influenced by his quiet and constant approach to art making as it helped me later, in my work with psychotic patients, to therapeutically frame an art studio and act as a nurturing presence in an open group (Deco, 1998; Wood, 2000). My memory is that Adamson suddenly left the art school in the middle of my one-year training. I can only guess that his 'non-interventionist' approach, which produced for me, and many of my peers, a tension between the freedom of non-verbal expression and a longing for recognition through spoken dialogue, was extensively challenged by the psychoanalytic ideas informing the education of art therapists nationally (Waller, 1991). In the wake of Adamson's departure, as students, we became members of a psychotherapy group, where no art was made. In the primarily verbal interactions of this group, and in the presence of a facilitator, new learning opened up about unconscious group processes that was in sharp contrast to the individual and private journeys embarked on in the open studio.

When I was appointed Art Therapy Programme Leader at the University of Hertfordshire in 1994, the course had evolved into a mature therapeutic training, firmly underpinned by psychodynamic theory. The earlier struggles of integrating psychoanalysis were superseded by the achievement of a symbiotic relationship with the School of Creative Arts: the creative milieu of the art school sustained the student's artistic practice, while the international reputation of the art therapy programme, its validation to MA level and HCPC status, afforded the School of Creative Arts much prestige. Despite this portfolio, below the surface of the institution lay a persistent ambivalence towards art therapy, initially voiced by Evans (cited in Waller, 1991: 236) who recognised that the art school experienced a threat to academic respectability when the word 'therapy' was attached to the fine arts. Elkins (2001: 44–45) debates how in teaching and learning art there is an osculation between the practice of art being a '*minimal coherent thing to do*' and a 'systematic intellectual pursuit', ideas that could be argued ironically mirror the academic journey of art therapy. An additional contributing factor to the ambivalence is a resistance towards a psychotherapeutic training, in the midst of an art school, that requires the extensive development of a student's emotional capacity, without which intellectual strivings in mastering concepts and theories are an empty endeavour (Symington, 1996: 11).

The studios and media workshops

The MA Art Therapy at the School of Creative Arts is successfully taught alongside contemporary postgraduate art and design courses. These disciplines, across the art school, share a premise that the studio creates the optimum conditions for a student's creative learning; it is in the studio that the student discovers process – the end goal of an exhibition or production of a product becomes secondary. The artist's studio is described by Buren and Repensek as 'the first frame, the first limit, upon which all subsequent frames/limits will depend' (1979: 51). These are the boundaries of walls and floor that allow experimentation and through its materiality traces the artists' working life (Sjöholm, 2013: 505). It could however be said that the traditional studio, in this contemporary and digital age, has become a misleading term as it has evolved into a site or location to be explored, with the work made somewhere else or by someone else. In terms of the studio as a learning space, it contributes to a recognition of status and commitment to an arts profession. Bain places particular emphasis on the relationship women artists have with the studio and how it 'functions as a powerful identity marker' (2004: 171–173) when historically women have been excluded from the male cannon of art history. Given the predominance of women training in art therapy, and the majority with first degrees in art and design, these ideas may have currency, with the studio a signifier of both artistic and therapeutic identity.

During my employment at the School of Creative Arts, I worked with many art therapy students who discovered they had entered a journey of artistic re-invention that held within it a recovery from the rigors of a previous art school education. In the context of experiential learning, this experience varied from those seeking a voice for personal struggles, kept at bay or overlooked at undergraduate level, to a resistance by others in letting go of a well-formed artistic identity. I discussed this complex process of artistic and personal resolution with a graduate, who described how returning to an art school as a trainee art therapist was loaded with paradox. Articulate in her reflections she acknowledged the attraction of the art school milieu, how it places art therapy in a wider visual cultural context and with a studio at her disposal the desire to paint had returned after a twenty-year gap. She was however unequivocal, about the 'unfinished business' of unravelling the critical edge of the institution, which had notably been previously manifest in a lack of reception to her introspective approach to art making.

The School of Creative Art has a number of well-equipped media workshops, which are a major attraction for students applying to the art therapy programme. These facilities of printmaking, sculpture, ceramics, and digital film allow postgraduate students, across all visual arts disciplines, to work alongside and extend their 'visual acuity' (Elkins, 2001: 103) into different art processes. In this expanded context of making and creating, art therapy students are exposed to the production of art outside the psychological frame of experiential learning. This shift, of reworking an image beyond the boundaries of its place of origin, heightens an awareness of the art therapy trainee's 'aesthetic response' to a thera-peutically intended artwork. In referencing the extensive body of literature on relational aesthetics and its relevance to service user's imagery in art therapy, Moon says as artists and art therapists an aesthetic response is 'not merely some-thing evoked in us as viewers, but is something we can actively engender by ways we respond to and engage with the artwork' (2002: 133–135). The process of creating a spontaneously handcrafted image, within the frame of the studio, then applying other processes in the media workshops was of particular benefit for stu-dents without a first degree in art. Entering under the 'special entry' criteria, many of these trainees acquired greater aesthetic and psychological attunement to the fabric of their own and the service user's process, with many newly identifying as painters, printmakers, or ceramic artists during their training.

Learning through studio practice

Buren and Repensek (1979) identify two specific types of studios, that of the European atelier based on the nineteenth-century system of apprenticeship and the American loft space exemplified by Warhol's The Factory in the 1960s. As traditions of the artist's studio these provide a history of individual artistic experi-mentation and collective collaborations. When bringing a psychological apprecia-tion of therapeutic space and its containment to this legacy, art therapists Andrea Gilroy and Mandy Rogers are representative. Gilroy speaks to how her inhibi-tions towards the 'affective content' of her artwork lessened as the boundaries between a 'super-ego lead studio-based fine artist' and the more 'libidinal urges of art therapy' became meaningless (2004: 73). Significantly, Rogers addresses how breaking the conventions of her painting and going outside the studio space lead to an 'observer self' (2002: 63) that deepened the connections she was able to make to the art of her elderly service users. On a postgraduate art therapy training, students follow their own artistic interests and are expected to understand a variety of media. This, coupled with the fact that the art therapy programme admits students from a broad spectrum of arts, humanity, and social science disciplines, sets up a range of expectations about how to engage in studio practice, individually and as a collective group of learners.

As a pivotal learning experience studio practice was loosely modelled on the 'open studio'; whereas in art therapy practice it is a 'reliable entity' (Deco, 1998: 101) that gives permission to the service user, in this instance, it allowed students to find themselves as an artist. At the start of the training, studio practice was broadly framed for students in terms of Winnicott's (1971) potential space, a secure base that could be playfully entered, left, and returned to as they chose. Encouragement was to inhabit the space with no expectation, beyond timetabled tutorials, to share artwork unless this happened naturally in pairs or small groups. Students were invited to learn from the freedom of having no formal tutor assessment, instead to reflect on connections between their own creative process and art therapy practice in a visual and written journal and termly tutorials. This private space, without assessment, was reported by students to be a liberation from a highly assessed course. When reminiscing, one graduate recalled the open studio as a place to muse and wonder. Another reflected on it being where all her 'imagining' of becoming an art therapist could take shape. Sjöholm (2013: 507) states that although the alchemy of the artistic process cannot always be completely revealed, the physical space of the studio leaves 'evidence' of something non-physical in ideas, thought, reflection, memory, or feeling intention. In this regard, it was noticeable from a tutor's perspective how the artistic, playful freedom of the open studio stirred concerns across the student body about revealing an inner self when faced with a blank sheet of paper, wall, or floor. In the context of learning to become attuned to a therapeutic process, these are tensions that provide an assimilation of art psychotherapeutic understanding, and service user experience, not purely as intellectual knowledge but through the artistic and 'emotional quest of the individual' (Symington, 1996: 21) on a visceral, temporal, and feeling level (Rogers, 2002: 60).

Like many art therapy students, the open studio was a conduit for a new experience of my art practice. Initially, I relished not having to engage with a visual narrative; for the first time, my art was allowed to be about nothing with little aesthetic value. At some point, I made a shift into the demands of the sculpture workshop. It was here, alongside the open studio, that I discovered a cross-fertilisation of materials and embodied expression and learnt how contexts elicit different meanings. In retrospective, I connect the endeavour to the work of German–American artist Eva Hesse (1936–1970), who transitioned from painting to sculpture in her short but illustrious career. Hesse described her process as 'non-art' seeing it as 'something and nothing' she understood that meaning arose circumstantially (Sussman, 2002: 31). This notion of nothingness in art making did not go unnoticed when many years later, as a tutor, I observed how in studio practice some students struggled with the desire for the open studio to deliver an 'Oceanic' (Freud, 2002) immersive experience, where artistic knowledge could be relinquished or an unearthing of talent discovered. More often, these unconscious wishes resulted in a sense of helplessness and being deskilled in the learner. However, pedagogically and psychotherapeutically, it could be argued that a parallel process such as this aids a trainee's understanding of the service users' regression in art therapy and provides a 'grounding effect' (Rogers, 2002: 69) in processing the psychological impact of the art therapeutic encounter.

Containment, identity, and dialogue

In her discussion on 'The Significance of Studios', Chris Wood names the art therapy studio as a 'second distinct level of containment . . . existing on the border between the therapist and the institution and the socio-political context'(Wood, 2000: 43). Learning the value of containment in relationship to a broad context of art therapy practices was played out in studio practice through absence. Students felt a loss of containment in the lack of storage provided to keep artwork safe and a timetable requirement to ritually return the studio to a neutral space. Questions about the flexibility of the boundaries of an open studio to contain were tested by the rubbish bins left overflowing or artwork abandoned and discarded. When images of particular significance were reported missing by the maker, followed by fruitless searches, this was cited as the institution not being a 'good enough' provider. Containment was felt to be illusive, across the student body, when artwork of rudimentary marks unwittingly revealed too much too quickly, and a tension built between a wish to be seen and a fear of exposure. Deco states that containment for the service user, in an open studio, consists of the opportunity for both 'interaction and withdrawal' (1998: 101). In this regard, some students retreated into sketch books or stayed away from the studio altogether to avoid the gaze of others. A graduate recalled how staying on the edge of the studio was a slow process of accepting herself as an artist, yet she said it significantly informed her art therapy practice 'being tentative and on the edge of the studio for a long time taught me the importance of waiting for the service user to come to art making. It forced me to be attuned to the non-verbal cues'.

Studio practice, without the constant gaze of a tutor, offers students less emotional constraint than a closed experiential group with a facilitator. In this instance, the more confident artists found a sense of belonging by bravely claiming the central performative space of the studio, effortlessly moving onto the walls, like hungry children they consumed the time and materials provided. Although the open studio invites a playful route to a new artistic identity, students have to tackle more infantile concerns of securing a place amongst peers. And, when issues alluding to authority or hierarchy raise themselves, one-to-one negotiation is a steep learning curve and in direct contrast to the experiential group, where power dynamics are addressed through the transference and held by the group leader.

While the discovery of a new artistic and therapeutic identity was, for the majority of art therapy students, rooted in the intimacy of the ongoing visual and verbal dialogues of experiential learning and placements, for some trainees it was the School of Creative Art's end-of-year exhibition that was most consolidating. Representing a wide variety of media and artistic approaches in art therapy, the curated space of the exhibition showcased a range of universal and personal themes, from attachment and loss, emerging identities, cultural difference, and the processing of service user experience. For one art therapy graduate the exhibition was a surprisingly significant event in her professional development. She recalled the experience of bringing her artwork out of the privacy of the studio into the public facing space of the exhibition, where amongst art and design disciplines, for the first time, she was rewarded by being seen as both artist and art therapist.

Further, learning from studio practice occurs in group tutorials where a triadic dialogue between observation, listening, and reflection takes place in the presence of a tutor. The tutor's role is not one of therapist but to facilitate the student's capacity to bring verbal language to their emerging art practice and hold a space where the therapeutic value of the open studio group dynamic can be acknowledged (Moon, 2002; Tripp, 2016). Tutorials create a space for students to share the range of media they use, from painting, drawing, installations, printmaking, and video and how these processes enable or inhibit therapeutic expression. Here, students learn to value and gain confidence in their own process of critical self-reflection and are awakened to how any avoidance of the matrix of relationships in the open studio may deprive them, and potentially the service user, of the experience of the capacity for 'being alone in the presence of someone' (Winnicott, 1971: 47), a central premise of the open studio model in practice. Additionally, tutorials keep an educational focus on the links art therapy has to the wider context of contemporary and modern art, with students encouraged to visit and appraise exhibitions in building a professional profile.

Conclusion

Moon's (2002: 53–54) idea that learning to help others communicate through the language of artistic expression comes from a deep immersion in art making while being exposed to the art of others is a strong argument in retaining the open studio experience on an art therapy training. The open studio has been a central and unique environment offered to service users in the history of the art therapy profession: for the art therapy student, studying in the milieu of an art school, it opens up a new artistically led journey that is personal, singular, and potentially collaborative. In relationship to the experiential groups, where the art therapy trainee's awareness of unconscious processes and interpersonal dynamics is heightened, the open studio allows the crossing of boundaries into other contexts and an exploration of the multiplicity of meaning in visual imagery. For the art therapy trainee, this process of migrating artwork, from one context to another, allows for previously learnt conventions in art practice to be broken down and a new authentic relationship discovered.

Although therapeutic knowledge and understanding about permissiveness, containment, witnessing, and personal revelation in art therapy is acquired across experiential learning, it is fundamentally bound up with the trainee's relationship to the 'first frame of the studio' (Buren and Repensek, 1979: 51) and the relational processes that occur within it. Educationally and fundamentally, it is the artistic freedom of personal expression afforded by the open studio that enables the art therapy student to make connections on a therapeutic and aesthetic level and bring the service user experience into sharp focus. These invaluable processes are supported by the broader context and legacy of art therapy at the School of Creative Arts, where an important interplay of visual acuity and symbolic understanding furthers the artistic and therapeutic identity of the art therapy trainee.

I would like to thank the following people:

Judy Glasman, former Dean, The School of Creative Arts, University of Hertfordshire, for sharing her work on the St Albans School of Art archive.
Graduates Rebecca Cox, Samantha Durant, and Emily Gray who generously discussed their learning experience of studio practice on the MA Art Therapy.

References

Bain, A. (2004) Female Artistic Identity in Place: The Studio. *Social and Cultural Geography*. 5 (2): 171–193.

Black Mountain College-A School Like No Other. TATESHOTS. (2016) www.tate.org.uk/art/art-terms/b/black-mountain-college/black-mountain-college-school-no-other (Accessed 9/11/2020).

Buren, D. and Repensek, T. (1979) *The Function of Studios*. October. Vol. 10 Autumn, 51–58. Cambridge, MA: MIT Press.

Davis, R. (2011) Are British Art Schools in Crisis as Fees Stifle a Creative Generation. *The Guardian*. www.theguardian.com/education/2011/oct/30/art-and-design-students-college-fees (Accessed 31/7/2020).

Deco, S. (1998) Return to the Open Studio Group: Art Therapy Groups in Acute Psychiatry. In *Art Psychotherapy Groups: Between Pictures and Words*. Skaife, S. and Huet, V. Eds. London: Routledge.

Elkins, J. (2001) *Why Art Can't be Taught*. Illinois: University of Illinois Press.

Freud, S. (2002) *Civilization and Its Discontents*. London: Penguin Books.

Gilroy, A. (2004) On Occasionally Being Able to Paint. *Inscape: The Journal of the British Association of Art Therapists*. 9 (2): 69–78.

Moon, C.H. (2002) *Studio Art Therapy: Cultivating the Artistic Identity of the Art Therapist*. London: Jessica Kingsley.

Rogers, M. (2002) Absent Figures: A Personal Reflection on The Value of Art Therapist's Own Image-Making. *Inscape: The Journal of the British Association of Art Therapists*. 7 (2): 59–71.

Sjöholm, J. (2013) The Art Studio as Archive: Tracing the Geography of Artistic Potentiality, Progress and Production. *Cultural Geographies in Practice* 21(3): 505–514.

St Albans School of Art Archive. (Accessed 2020).

Sussman, E. (ed.) (2002) *Eva Hesse*. San Francisco: Museum of Modern Art, Yale University Press.

Symington, N. (1996) *The Making of a Psychotherapist*. London: Karnac Books.

Tripp, S. (2016) Reflections on the Evolving Triad Tutorial in a Postgraduate Art Studio. *The International Journal of Art and Design Education*. 35 (3): 384–394.

Waller, D. (1991) *Becoming a Profession: The History of Art Therapy in Britain 1940–82*. London, Tavistock/Routledge.

Winnicott, D. (1971) *Playing and Reality*. London: Penguin Books.

Wood, C. (2000) The Significance of Studios. *Inscape: The Journal of the British Association of Art Therapists*. 5 (2): 40–52.

7 Studio encounters

A personal view of shifting frames in art therapy

Christopher Brown

Introduction

What is a studio? It is a dedicated space. What it is dedicated to may vary according to whatever media is involved. It should be free from the impingements of daily living activities and thus be a space apart from them. In an art studio, the availability of art materials allows engagement with creative expression. It may be important that there is room to move around and to make a mess. These requirements apply to the art therapy studio also but with an important addition, that of the therapist who facilitates the use of the space by others. The specialised setting of the art therapy studio can enable provision not only of a space to engage in creative expression through art but also, within a psychodynamic framework of thinking, can be understood as offering people experiences of a holding environment (Winnicott, 1965) and containment (Bion, 1967) as aspects of the maternal function (Chasseguet-Smirgel, 1984). These are essentially non-verbal aspects of experience. In art therapy, the art is made in the context of a relationship and the setting is part of the relationship, not something separate from it (Brown, 2008). The relationship may be foregrounded when working with transference or be part of the background in studio-based approaches where the art is the focus.

This chapter draws upon my personal history as an art therapist in the National Health Service (NHS) to explore the effect of different contexts within which my work and interests have been framed and how this influenced my ideas about art therapy studios. These contexts comprise complex interactions between the social, cultural, and political spheres, which means that clear distinctions may not always be possible.

Two contexts were driven by government legislation concerning the care for the mentally ill. The first of these was the Lunacy Act of 1890, which placed an obligation on local authorities to maintain institutions for the mentally ill, which resulted in the establishment of many of the Victorian asylums where the pioneers of art therapy worked. The second was the 1990 NHS and Community Care Act, which saw the large-scale closure of the old asylums and provision for locally based services integrated into the communities they served. A third came about through the rise of neoliberalism and its impact on the way that public sector services such as the NHS are run. The basic idea underpinning neoliberalism, as

DOI: 10.4324/9781003095606-9

formulated by the economist Friedman, is 'that when businesses are left alone to get on with making money for themselves, then not only will the businesses flourish, so will the economy, and this will be of benefit to society as a whole' (Dalal, 2018: 77). As a consequence, the concept of managed care was imported from the US healthcare system and adopted by the new NHS managers who were brought in to implement the policy.

Another context that influenced the frame of my art therapy practice was psychoanalysis. In 1999, I undertook a personal analysis that was to last thirteen years. Alongside this, I gained a master's degree in the foundations of psychoanalytic psychotherapy at the Tavistock Centre in London, which was essentially a psychotherapy training involving the close supervision of a training patient but not a qualification to practice as a psychotherapist. It did, however, enable me to work with transference when I felt this was appropriate, and it clarified my commitment to practice as an art therapist and not to change horses midstream and become a psychotherapist. Feeling secure to practice art therapy within a psychodynamic framework was central to my work, not only in extended exploratory treatments but also in more studio-based work, where an understanding of unconscious phenomena such as projective identification and countertransference were important in providing containment.

My social context changed when I retired from working in the NHS and became a freelancer. This seemed to free up my thinking and led me to explorations outside of my usual frames of reference pertaining to clinical work. A number of linked projects came about in a short space of time that made me rethink the framing of art in art therapy. I made a film about an Arts in Health project undertaken by Errol Fernandes some years previously. Errol had been employed as an artist on the project, but he was also a practising art therapist. In producing the film together, we had many interesting discussions on how far you can stretch the frame before it is no longer deemed to be art therapy. Also, I came to know the work of Studio Upstairs, who were a partner in the original Arts in Health project. I saw an exhibition at the New Art Studio, a therapeutic art studio for refugees and asylum seekers in London, which led to a number of recorded discussions with two colleagues about what happens when you take the art out of the art therapy frame. This project eventually led to a jointly written review of an exhibition of selected works from the Edward Adamson Collection (Brown et al., 2017).

My internal compass had shifted and was now pointing in a different direction and another journey beckoned towards thinking about the differing frameworks of art therapy practice. In particular, I wanted to think through in what ways the context in which the frame sits defines the boundaries of the frame.

Beginnings

My first encounter with a dedicated art therapy studio, as a professional art therapist, was when I started work at Hill End Hospital, Hertfordshire in 1991. This was an old-style asylum built in 1899. The art therapy department there was an extraordinary space created out of what had previously been a hospital ward. It

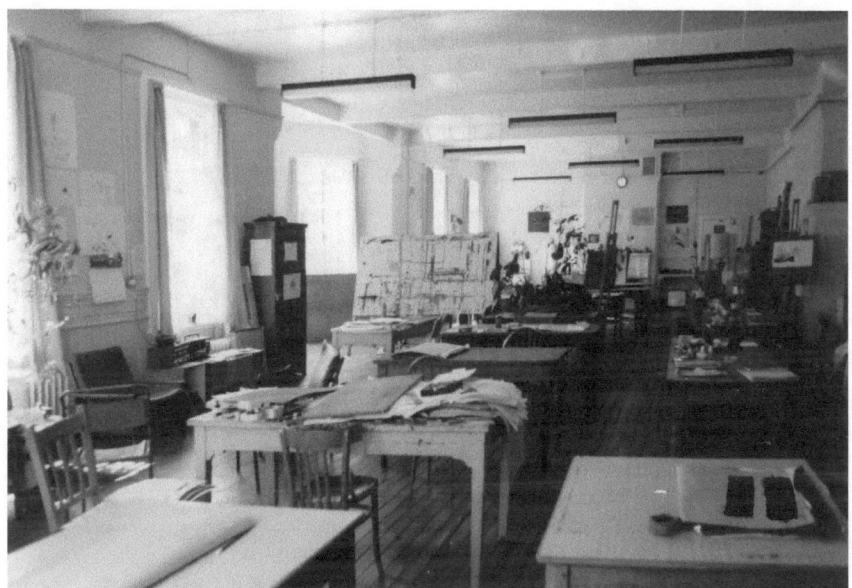

Figure 7.1

was set up as a large studio with individual table space allocated to each patient. The layout, as shown in Figure 7.1, was established by Katherine Killick according to her ideas about working with patients in acute psychotic states (Killick, 1993, 2000). Being with people experiencing psychosis was a shock to my system. Ordinary relating was rarely possible, more often it was a cacophony of fragmented utterances, weird looks, and difficult behaviour that I did not know how to manage but had to tolerate somehow while in the studio. These encounters with fragmented minds threatened the capacity of my own mind to contain what they evoked and on occasion this found expression through my own art making. Figure 7.2 shows a decorative banner that I made for a Christmas party for patients held in the department around that time. There was a sense of freedom from restriction that I experienced there while simultaneously feeling I was walking a tightrope over a pit of seething snakes.

Over time, I began to understand how the studio functioned as a 'place for the mind to heal' (Killick, 2017: 3). Before this can happen 'the traumatic threat that the relationship with the therapist presents' (Ibid.: 3) needs to be negotiated. This requires an appreciation of the loss of the symbolising function in psychosis and the associated concrete nature of thinking and feeling, along with the use of the art making process and product as an intermediary object within the relationship (Killick, 1993). Negotiations around the artwork and the studio setting involving both concrete and psychic space help reduce psychotic anxieties. In this way, the therapeutic relationship acquires a more benign quality, and the studio can start to

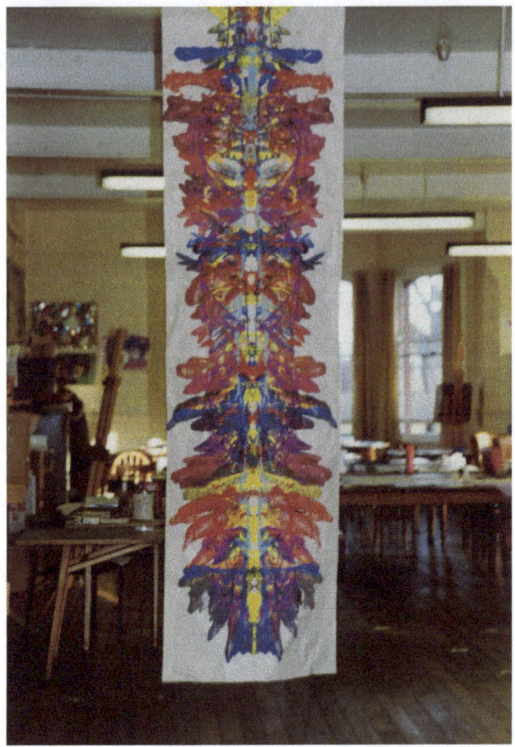

Figure 7.2

function as a healing agent. For example, when a patient asked to put a picture up in the studio I was able to offer him an entire wall (Brown, 2008). He periodically changed the pictures, and I would help in getting them positioned as he wished. This collaborative curating gave expression to the value of the art, of him, and of the relationship.

The therapist's state of mind and the part it plays in projective processes that may be encountered in the studio setting are also important. The idea that non-verbal communication predominates in encounters with psychosis has been explored by the psychoanalyst Herbert Rosenfeld (1987). Such communication is often experienced as an emotionally charged atmosphere that may lead the therapist to feel overwhelmed or act in particular ways in response. If the therapist is able to pick up on such disturbing entanglements and respond with empathy this will be felt by the other person as a benign rather than malign encounter. In general, it is the attitude and behaviour of the therapist that communicates this empathy and contributes to the establishment of the studio as a holding environment. It took me some time before I was able to put these ideas into practice effectively – it was in another studio that this happened and to which I now turn.

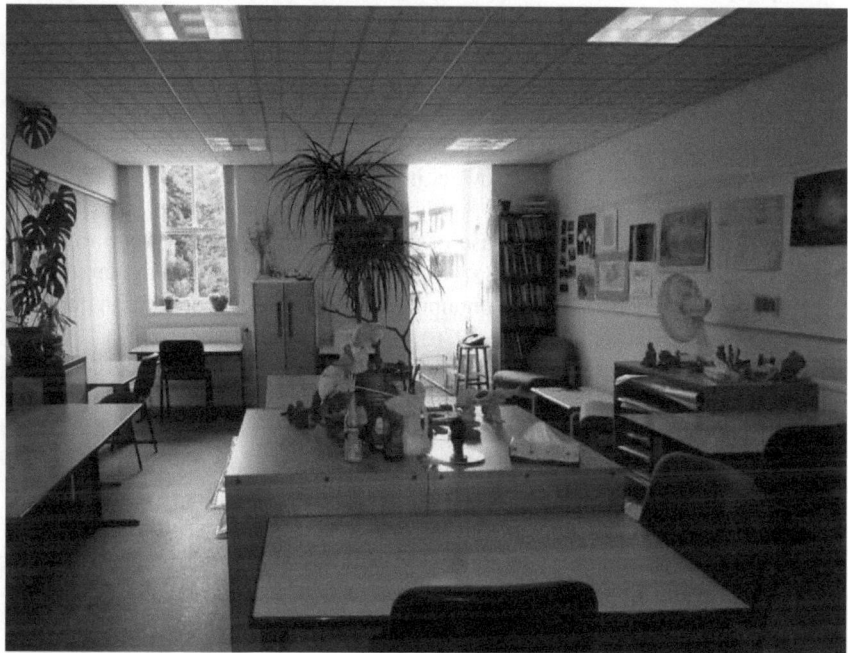

Figure 7.3

Changes

Five years later, in 1996, this art therapy department moved to a new location away from the hospital and into the community as a result of the NHS and Community Care Act (1990). This change in the context in which the frame of the art therapy service sat had a number of consequences. We no longer saw people in such acute psychotic states due to the studio's distant location from the new group homes and unavailability of nursing staff. Instead, we saw a broader psychiatric population. Also, we developed closer liaison with the Community Mental Health Team (CMHT), which included an expanding psychotherapy department.

We were given a delightful old building in the middle of the town. The art therapy department had to share this with a Day Centre – providing support and activities – and the Dramatherapy service. We were able to specify our need for a dedicated art therapy studio, as a discreet space, separate and clearly boundaried from the other services using the building. There were times when we came under pressure to allow others access to our studio space, but this was always resisted. Our need for a dedicated, confidential space, and willingness to defend it, was perhaps envied by others. The space was large enough not to feel too claustrophobic yet small enough to feel cosy when making art and sitting talking (see Figure 7.3). The studio was used for individual and group art therapy. In addition, on two half-days a week the space became an open studio for selected patients who could use an extended time period in which to make art. This time was facilitated by an art therapist from the team who would be responsible for the space during those hours. However, each of these patients was also seen separately, at a different time, and perhaps in a different room, by their personal therapist to discuss their work. In this way and at those times in the week the studio function echoed that of early pioneers, such as Champernowne, in separating the process of making and the exploration of content.

In an article that looked at the use of art making in the studio from an object relations perspective (Brown, 2008), I drew upon concepts such as the facilitating environment (Winnicott, 1965), containment (Bion, 1967), countertransference, and role responsiveness (Sandler, 1976) in order to think about the non-verbal aspects of the therapeutic relationship. My understanding of the five-year long therapy with a man diagnosed with schizophrenia, which I described, was clearly from a psychoanalytic perspective.

Another example highlights the potential for a more socially oriented aspect of studio art therapy. This man, who I will call Stephen, had a psychotic break-down while studying astrophysics at university and was now in his sixties. He was referred due to concerns about his increasing social isolation and his paranoid delusions; the aim of treatment was to prevent deterioration resulting from his withdrawn states of mind. Stephen had weekly access to one of the open studio sessions described earlier, and I saw him for a separate thirty-minute meeting every two weeks over a seven-year period. In our conversations any comment on the content of his pictures quickly spiralled out of control and into his delusory system of flying saucers and media manipulations. Instead, we focussed on his art, which we spoke about in terms of their aesthetic qualities. In general, I kept any thoughts about what they might mean to myself but over time he did start to mention things that happened to him in his life, both past and present. I responded to these communications in an everyday sort of way that acknowledged his lived experience with empathy and respect. In this way, an alliance was formed between us whereby I tried to remain non-intrusive, and he tried to let me into his life, little by little. This gave him an experience of conviviality that I believe helped him to relate at a deeper level than his only other social contact – his weekly super-market shop. Wood highlights this aspect: 'There is some tension between the psychological need for private protected space (or containment) and the notion of *convivencia* (mingling), but essentially sharing and fruitful exchange seems to depend upon the availability of a *good* containing environment' (2010: 9).

Three of his pictures are shown here. The first (Figure 7.4) is from early on and depicts a barren landscape overlaid with what he called a 'net' within which is the word 'Voideo' – a pun on void and video. The second (Figure 7.5) depicts three flying saucers. The third (Figure 7.6) contains the repeated motif of the three flying saucers but in a newly emerging style some years later following a change from using marker pens to coloured pencils. Here, the curving shapes are reminiscent of leaves, suggesting growth, and are in contrast to the barren rocks depicted previously.

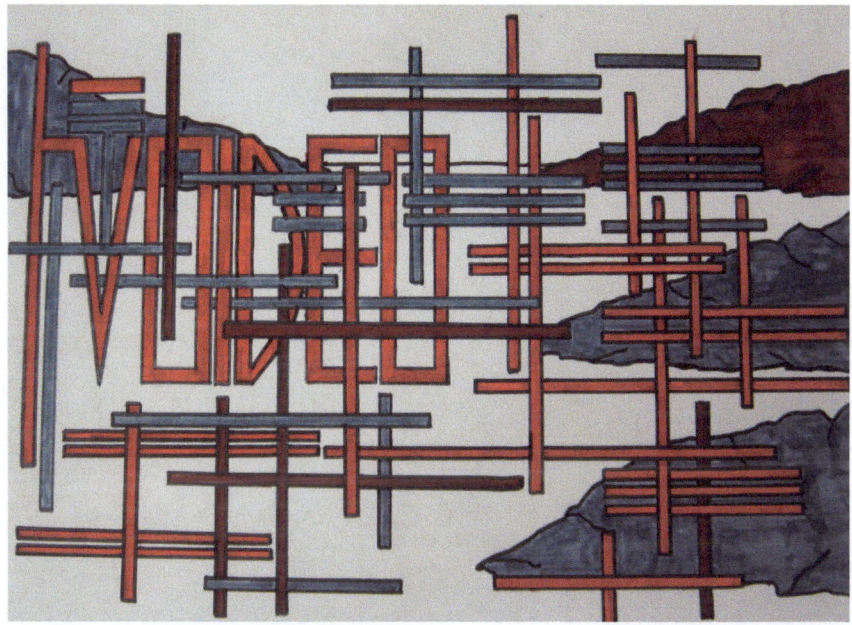

Figure 7.4

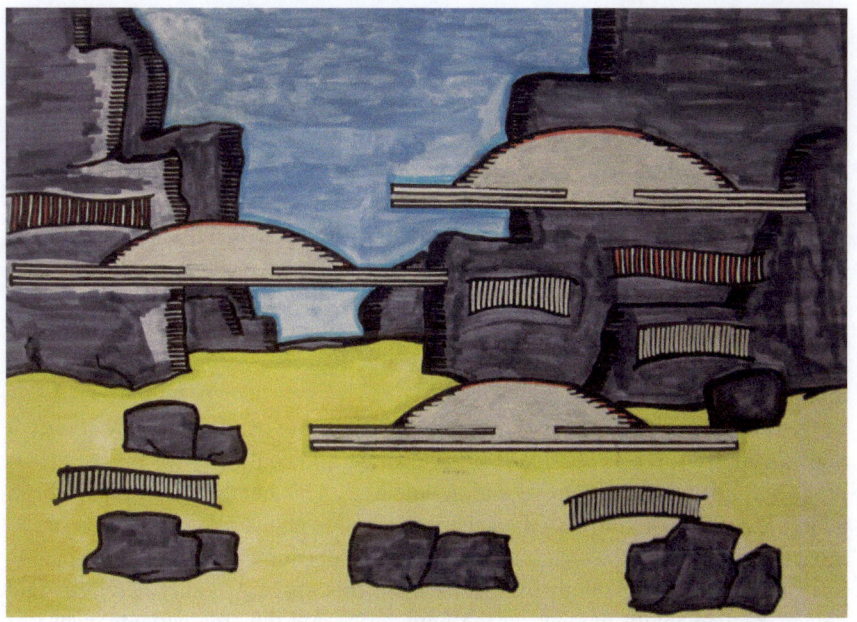

Figure 7.5

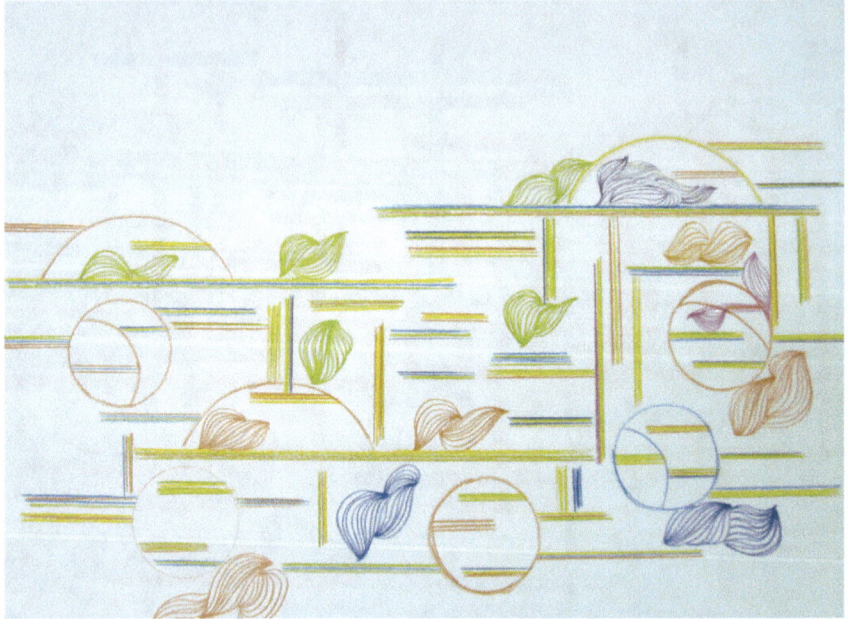

Figure 7.6

The lost studio

Managed care is a term used to describe the US healthcare system, which aims to provide cost-effective treatments with outcomes that can be measured and set against targets. In the UK, recent government initiatives and reorganisation have brought managed care more fully into the NHS. In this context, cost-effectiveness resulted in the closure of the building in which the studio described earlier was housed and a move into the local Community Mental Health Centre (CMHC) in 2012. Furthermore, it meant we had to share a room with dramatherapy colleagues. We quickly discovered how our needs differed from theirs and learnt about the dogma of multi-use rooms. Our new manager, a drama therapist, was against us putting any pictures up on the walls. Figure 7.7 shows the bareness of this space.

There are very good reasons for maintaining sole use of an art therapy studio. It allows a high degree of confidentiality, security, and continuity for the art that is produced, displayed, and stored within the space. This holding function has been an integral part of studio-based art therapy practice and is often crucial in allowing engagement with the creative and therapeutic encounters we provide to people in disturbed states of mind. Intrusions upon this space by other activities and objects fundamentally impact on the boundaries and thus the patients' sense of feeling sufficiently 'held' by this space. This might equally apply to the therapist,

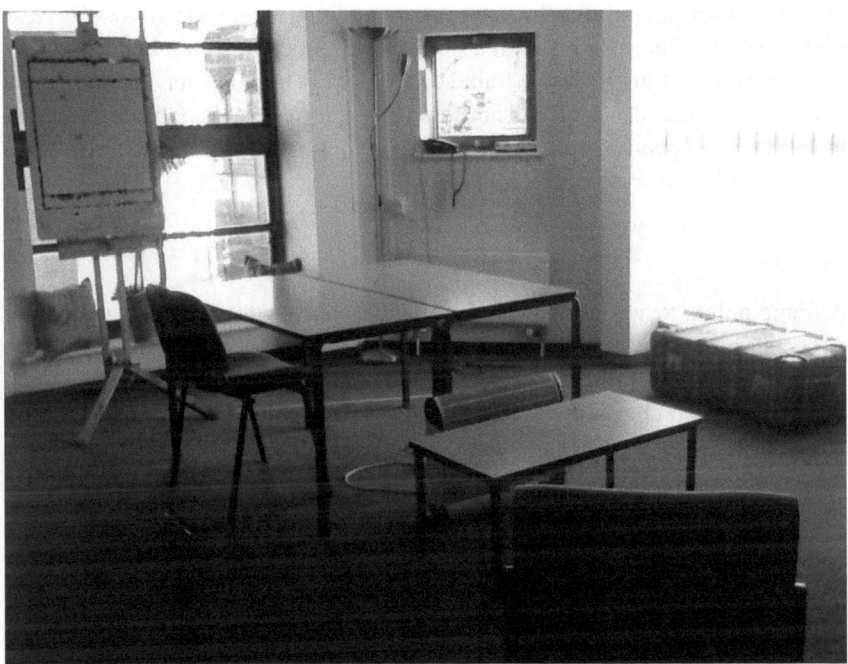

Figure 7.7

who requires a secure setting in which the exposure to emotional turmoil can be contained (see Brown, 2014 for an example of this).

I felt this change of setting as a loss, hence the heading for this section – 'The lost studio' – which was also the title of a paper I presented at the International Art Therapy conference in 2013 (Ibid.). It had a subtitle 'You don't know what you've got till it's gone' taken from a Joni Mitchell song and the line continues 'they paved paradise, put up a parking lot' (1970). This sentiment echoes my feelings about the loss of suitable studio spaces for long-term involvements in art therapy. The loss of such studios has increased under ideological demands that require the bland orderliness of efficient but insipid spaces rather than humanised ones with their sensory tang and patina of living.

Perhaps this loss of a dedicated studio was the crucial experience for me. One that took me into a mourning process where I was seeking to regain what was lost. It can be hard to know how shifts in one's thinking occur. Certainly, the changes taking place in the NHS Trust, in large part due to the government's 'payment by results' policy (Department of Health, 2012), during my last year there left me feeling restricted in my clinical art therapy practice and I was glad to leave when the opportunity presented itself through reaching retirement age. What followed was a development of my ideas about art therapy through the continuation of my teaching on trainings; writing articles and editorial work for the open access, online journal *ATOL*: *Art Therapy OnLine*; and developing my own art practice. Being able to think more widely about the context in which the frame of art therapy practice may sit helped me to understand the reasons for the different boundaries that may be encountered in various therapeutic art studios – both those described earlier and those I was now becoming interested in.

Frames

A frame points to what is inside, forming a boundary to what it contains, but also relates to what is outside – the context in which it sits. It is this context that influences the construction of the frame. For example, the context in which Edward Adamson began his work at Netherne Hospital was one of psychiatric research. This dictated how his studio was set up and the materials available for use by patients, whose work was subsequently presented to the psychiatrists Cunningham-Dax and Reitman for their analysis (Cunningham-Dax, 1953; Reitman, 1950). Once this research ended, he had more freedom to run the studio according to his own principles of artistic expression and art education (Adamson, 1984).

The context for my work in the art therapy department at Hill End Hospital was both the legacy of the approach used by Katherine Killick and the practice of psychiatric care for the mentally ill as performed by the institution. From this, I constructed what I now think of as a 'shaky' frame for my own practice of art therapy. One in which I was never quite sure if I knew what I was doing or not.

The move from institutional location to a community one brought with it a greater sense of autonomy for me that allowed the development of my own approach to the work. Whilst this was informed by psychoanalytic ideas, the daily involvement with the art therapy studio kept me thinking about the nature of this space and the art making processes it contained.

The eventual loss of this community studio and a new freelance role led to encounters with frames of art therapy practice that prompted further thinking about the studio art therapy approach. For example, my supervision of art therapists working with the homeless and with an organisation set up in response to the Grenfell tower disaster (see Rudnik, 2018). In doing so, I started to realise that a lot of what I was seeing and hearing about reminded me of ideas that were part of my own cultural influences in the 1960s – ideas about social equality, destigmatisation of mental illness, challenging of the establishment, and freedom of expression. The development of art therapy studios during that period of experimentation and social change in the 1960s drew upon ideas from the antipsychiatry movement, phenomenology, and therapeutic communities – ideas that we are still processing today.

In 1962, the psychiatrist David Cooper set up Villa 21 at Shenley Hospital with a non-hierarchical approach to working with young male schizophrenics (Cooper, 1970). In summing up the development of the unit, he says:

> During the four years of the unit's life we have progressively and successfully eliminated many destructive aspects of psychiatric institutional life. We have eliminated formal hierarchization to a point beyond which no similar experiment in the literature of the subject has gone.
>
> (1970: 112)

Although this experiment closed after four years, his ideas about therapeutic communities were to find another, perhaps more radical, home. Cooper, along with fellow psychiatrist R.D. Laing, was a founding member of the Philadelphia Association, which became synonymous with antipsychiatry and new ways of perceiving mental illness. They were both interested in existential philosophy and psychoanalysis and provided 'asylum' in community households for people suffering mental distress. Cooper again:

> [W]e have arranged through personal contact for some discharged patients to live with reliable people (i.e. non-mystifying, minimally anxious people) in houses in the community in small groups. These projects . . . present the best and most creative alternative to the stultifying or even untenable position that the patient gets into in his family home and in the institution.
>
> (1970: 113/4)

It was such community households that offered embodied lived experience in the company of others in which the concept of 'dwelling' was central. Robin Cooper puts it thus: 'By this, I refer to a *way* of being with one another and knowing one's way in the world which is *being at home*' (1989: 42, italics in original). Therapeutic art studios offer similar experience where people may 'dwell' for periods of time in their life.

The ideas and understandings of the causes and treatment of mental illness that came from the antipsychiatry movement (Szasz, 1961; Laing, 1960, 1967) struggled against the rising tide of the biomedical model and advances in the neurosciences that followed. In setting out the main argument of his book, *Doctoring The Mind: Is our current treatment of madness really any good?*, Richard Bentall says:

> What has been lost in all this is that it might be possible to be rationally antipsychiatric, that conventional psychiatry might reasonably be criticised, not on hard-to-define humanistic grounds (although these are important) but because it has been profoundly unscientific and at the same time unsuccessful at helping some of the most distressed and vulnerable people in our society.
>
> (2009: xvii)

He goes on to add 'if psychiatric services are to become more generally therapeutic, and if they are to help people rather than merely 'manage' their difficulties, it will be necessary to rediscover the art of relating to patients with warmth, kindness and empathy' (2009: xix). It seems that things have not changed much in the forty years between the critiques of David Cooper and Richard Bentall.

What then may constitute the elements that make up the frame within which studio art therapy can be viewed? I think, first and foremost, it is the provision of a particular kind of space. Robin Cooper suggests:

> Space is not some ether which surrounds and envelops us, but a field of openings and depths held or subtended by vectors of intentionality. The example of a sportsman upon his field of play, or a dancer upon the floor, may illustrate quite well that lived spatiality, that freedom of movement, which belongs with 'being at home'.
>
> (1989: 43)

Institutions tend to close down spaces, offering little room to breathe and move, rather they coerce and dehumanise the people who inhabit them. Art therapy studios offer an alternative space, one that allows movement between private and public space. The space may be completely open in that anyone can enter or there may be gatekeeping functions such as referral and assessment, but once in the space there is usually a freedom to come and go on your own terms. Work may happen in corners, on easels, or the walls. Having the space to move around may be more comfortable than the fixed circle of analytic groups. Lessening the intensity of the encounter – the persecutory anxiety of examination – can be key to engagement.

Being seen and seeing oneself as a person making art is very different to seeing oneself as a patient or client receiving treatment or a service. The making of art is seen as a primary focus in studio art therapy. The therapist may focus on the aesthetic qualities of the work, as an art teacher might, or encourage experimentation with art materials. Work may be exhibited in a gallery. Alongside this fostering of artistic identity are interactions concerned more with processes and materials than eliciting meaning for psychological insight. Discussion about materials may be seen concretely by the person using them or by the therapist as a way to modify, for example, tendencies to rigidity or looseness in personality addressed through the intermediary of the materials rather than directly to the person. There is a paradigm shift in the way of relating by the therapist, who seeks to establish a non-intrusive engagement reflecting the benign presence of another, which is so different from the relentless questioning often found in other clinical encounters.

Conclusion

A studio offers its user a particular kind of space, one that is apart from everyday life where creative activity can be discovered. The primary focus of the endeavour is the making of art. Life in the studio offers a way of being with one another that might be described as akin to dwelling, a feeling of being at home (Cooper et al., 1989). The Hill End Hospital studio developed a frame suited to working with people in psychotic states of mind where clear boundaries were crucial. Here I learnt how stirred up the therapist's state of mind can become when exposed to the unconscious use of primitive mechanisms of defence for communication. Also, it gave me an experience of a space that could contain such states of mind. The institution still loomed large, for me at least, with a somewhat antiquated psychiatric ideology. The move into a community-based studio brought a consolidation of those elements and a period of personal stability that enabled me to develop different approaches. One based on the use of the studio with the focus on making art, the other on use of the therapeutic relationship and a focus on unconscious conflicts. With the loss of this particular studio and a move into a much 'colder' clinical space in the CMHC, I felt squeezed into a frame that did not support the elements of my approach to art therapy that I had come to value.

This particular frame arose out of what Farhad Dalal, in his book *CBT: The Cognitive Behavioural Tsunami* (2018), calls the holy trinity of 'psychological science, neoliberalism and managerialism', within which psychological treatments are being forced to operate. In referring to the particular ideology within which psychological science has located itself in the NHS, he says: 'Hyper-rationality is the use of a reductive version of rationality in contexts that are not suited to it' (2018: 3). Hyper-rationality insists the evidence-base for treatments must 'be only of the arithmetic kind, because numbers and measurements are objective and real. If something can't be counted, if it cannot be measured, *then it does not exist; it is not real*' (Ibid., italics in original). He goes on to demonstrate how the marketisation of services leads to ever-narrower parameters being applied to the kind and duration of therapy available in the NHS. It seems to me that something valuable has been lost in this process – the value of what we deem to be ethical and meaningful in our interactions with human suffering – which art therapy studios have been providing for the past eighty years.

The context within which the frame sits inevitably changes according to the shifts in social, political, and cultural spheres that reflect developmental processes for humankind. The current context is one where collective anxieties arising from those processes lead to the tendency towards binary thinking and opposing ideologies. What Bollas (2021) calls pathological group thinking as an understandable psychotic, social process – one that we need to understand in order to change people's way of thinking. We are living in extraordinary times. Climate change and environmental destruction may lead politicians to make radical changes in the economics of neoliberalism and the pursuit of corporate profit. Our social infrastructure is being broken down by such policies and the value of community is in danger of being lost. Perhaps it is time for a fundamental reordering of social priorities, one that shifts the balance back to the utopian ideals that studio art therapy contains. We need both preservation and innovation.

Acknowledgement

This chapter draws upon a conference paper previously published in *ATOL: Art Therapy OnLine* Vol 5 No 1 (2014).

References

Adamson, E. (1984) *Art as Healing*. London: Coventurer.

Bentall, R. P. (2009) *Doctoring the Mind: Is Our Current Treatment of Madness Really Any Good?* London: Allen Lane.

Bion, W. R. (1967) *Second Thoughts*. London: Heinemann.

Bollas, C. (2021) Civilization and the discontented. In *Psychoanalysis and Covidian Life: Common Distress, Individual Experience*, edited by Howard B. Levine and Ana Staal. Bicester, Oxfordshire: Phoenix Publishing House.

Brown, C. (2008) Very toxic – Handle with care. Some aspects of the maternal function in art therapy. *International Journal of Art Therapy*, 13(1): 13–24.

———. (2014) The lost studio: "You don't know what you've got till it's gone". *ATOL: Art Therapy OnLine*, 5(1). Available at: http://journals.gold.ac.uk/index.php/atol/article/view/345/375.

Brown, C., Martyn, J. and Skaife, S. (2017) Exhibition review: Mr A moves in mysterious ways: Selected artists from the Adamson collection, Peltz gallery, Birkbeck school of arts, 15th May to 25th July 2017. *ATOL: Art Therapy OnLine*. Available at: http://journals.gold.ac.uk/index.php/atol/article/view/464/pdf.

Chasseguet-Smirgel, J. (1984) The femininity of the analyst in professional practice. *International Journal of Psycho-Analysis*, 65: 169–178.

Cooper, D. (1970) *Psychiatry and Anti-Psychiatry*. St Albans, Herts: Paladin.

Cooper, R., Gans, S., Heaton, J. M., Oakley, H. and Zeal, P. (1989) Beginnings. In *Thresholds between Philosophy and Psychoanalysis: Papers from the Philadelphia Association*, edited by R. Cooper et al. London: Free Association Books.

Cunningham-Dax, E. (1953) *Experimental Studies in Psychiatric Art*. London: Faber and Faber.

Dalal, F. (2018) *CBT: The Cognitive Behavioural Tsunami. Managerialism, Politics, and the Corruption of Science*. London: Routledge.

Department of Health. (2012) *A Simple Guide to Payment by Results*. London: DOH.

Killick, K. (1993) Working with psychotic processes in art therapy. *Psychoanalytic Psychotherapy*, 7(1): 25–38.

———. (2000) The art room as container in analytical art psychotherapy with patients in psychotic states. In *The Changing Shape of Art Therapy*, edited by A. Gilroy and G. McNeilly. London: Jessica Kingsley, pp. 99–114.

———. (2017) Places for the mind to heal. In: *Art Therapy for Psychosis: Theory and Practice*, edited by Katherine Killick. London: Routledge.

Laing, R. D. (1960) *The Divided Self*. London: Tavistock Press.

———. (1967) *The Politics of Experience and the Bird of Paradise*. London: Penguin.

Mitchell, J. (1970) *Big Yellow Taxi*, from the album Ladies of the Canyon. New York: Warner Records Inc.

Reitman, F. (1950) *Psychotic Art*. London: Routledge.

Rosenfeld, H. (1987) *Impasse and Interpretation*. London: Tavistock Publications.

Rudnik, S. (2018) Out of the darkness: A community led art psychotherapy response to the Grenfell tower fire. *ATOL: Art Therapy OnLine*, 9(1). Available at: http://journals.gold.ac.uk/index.php/atol/article/view/491/pdf.

Sandler, J. (1976) Countertransference and Role-responsiveness. *International Review of Psycho-analysis*: 43–7.

Szasz, T. S. (1961) *The Myth of Mental Illness*. New York: Harper and Row.

Winnicott, D. W. (1965). *The Maturational Process and the Facilitating Environment*. London: The Hogarth Press.

Wood, C. (2010) Convivencia: A medieval idea with contemporary relevance. *ATOL: Art Therapy OnLine*, 1(1). Available at: http://journals.gold.ac.uk/index.php/atol/article/view/218/233.

Part II
Models of practice

8 The Community Table

Developing art therapy studios on, in-between, and across borders

Bobby Lloyd and Miriam Usiskin

Introduction

This chapter explores The Community Table as an evolving model of practice originating in a context of crisis support. It has developed from initial beginnings at a dining room table in a safe house for young unaccompanied refugees. When working in the border town of Calais, northern France, the lack of consistent safe spaces has required a clear rationale for the work and adaptations to models, which have roots in the art therapy studio. The Community Table can be metaphorically concertinaed to expand, or contract. It has supported a dynamic way of working on, in-between, and across borders, real and symbolic. This model has been translated by Art Refuge to other settings including online under COVID-19. It opens up possibilities for thinking about art therapy studios in settings that previously may have felt out of reach.

The chapter presents four iterations of The Community Table. One was developed in response to the COVID-19 pandemic. The political and social context, seasons and weather, location and spaces available, and the displaced demographic present shaped each manifestation. This in turn informed what art materials and media were introduced.

The work described was undertaken by the charity Art Refuge which supports the mental health and well-being of people displaced due to conflict, persecution, and poverty in the UK and internationally. Offering specialist art and art therapy spaces, its team of visual artists and art therapists includes a growing number of artists with lived experience as refugees.

In order to reach the UK to claim asylum, refugees have gathered since the late 1990s in the France–UK border town of Calais, where the route across the English Channel to Dover is at its shortest. The vast majority have been men. With almost no safe or legal routes available, men, as well as women, children, and families, have taken desperate risks to cross the Channel in trains, trucks, and most recently in small boats, often aided by networks of smugglers and traffickers. Since 2015 Art Refuge has operated in the Calais area. Its team has frequently witnessed human rights violations in the form of endemic violence perpetrated by French state police, regular clearances of makeshift camps, and restrictions on basic amenities including access to shelter, food, drinking water, and showers.

DOI: 10.4324/9781003095606-11

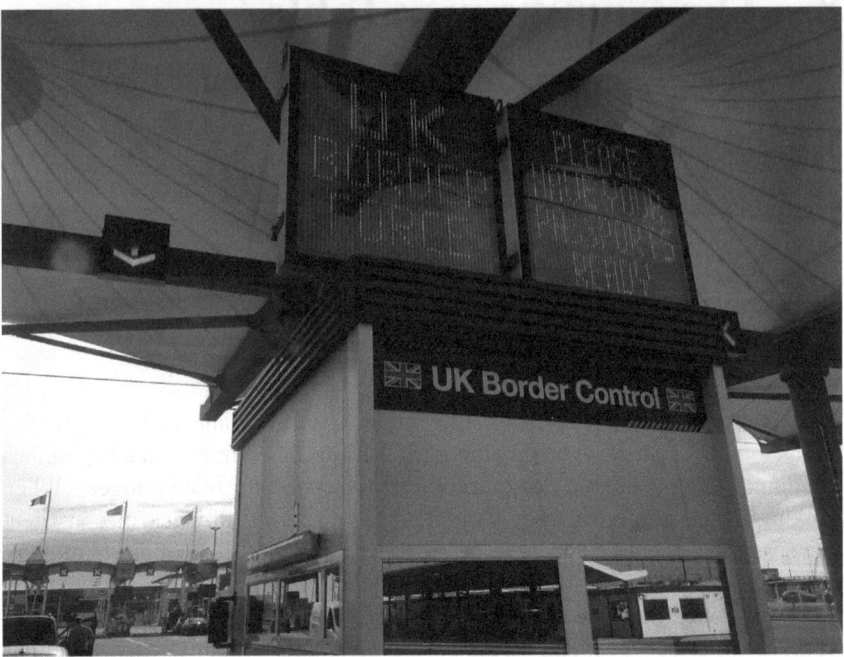

Figure 8.1 UK border control.

This policy has been supported by the British government, which has invested millions of pounds of public funds on border control in Calais and the surrounding area, including the visible construction of numerous walls and fences.

Refugees stuck on the border have been supported by French and British non-government organisations (NGOs). Operating alongside Médecins du Monde and Secours Catholique up until the closing of the border in March 2020 due to COVID-19, Art Refuge worked in a variety of settings: makeshift refugee settlements, a state-recognised camp, day centres, a mobile clinic, roadsides, a petrol station, an apartment, a homeless hostel, and a safe house. Its team supported hundreds of male refugees, many of whom were teenagers, running bimonthly psychosocial art and art therapy spaces.

Developing partnerships at the invitation of the two main French humanitarian organisations in Calais was a deliberate choice so as to provide Art Refuge with local infrastructure and knowledge. This gave access to workspace, storage, interpreters, multidisciplinary team meetings, risk, and safeguarding protocols – all essential to keep the work safe and grounded. It has led to rich collaborations sustained over a number of years and ongoing at the time of writing, with Art Refuge also offering training and skills-sharing for other organisations working on the ground.

From the early days the team realised that, for refugees in transit, mobile phones are often their only possession, while social media can offer a route through which connections can be maintained and information found and shared. Enabling a voice for those who are disaffected and marginalised has been manifested through the charity's use of social media.

Contextual and theoretical framework

Studio art therapy

Kapitan (2008) describes therapeutic art studios as being places where community transformation can happen through a collective dynamic, often taking place with marginalised groups and in unconventional settings, such as disaster relief. These therapeutic studios can move away from a one-dimensional model that includes the treatment of pathology towards a more progressive stance: 'Something happens when the narrative of the profession shifts from the individual expert to the living reality and power of the collective' (Kapitan, 2008: 2).

Nolan (2019) explores the mechanisms that influence change in the Community Art Therapy Studio, which she defines as a co-created space made by users of the service as well as facilitators. She identifies that there is a role for art therapists to use their knowledge and skills in an improvised way: 'a here and now manner that responds to the actions and interactions of the studio participants and is not prescribed' (Nolan, 2019: 78). This idea, alongside the notions of a 'not knowing' stance (Anderson, 1997) and 'disciplined improvisation' (Crane et al., 2014) brings together a rigorous approach that supports The Community Table with the recognition of the inherent demands for flexible adaptation to situations beyond our control.

Given the volatile context, The Community Table model is akin to Moon's mobile art therapy studio. She describes this as

> a far cry from the idealised image most people have of a quiet studio environment, a sanctuary set apart from the rest of life. Instead, it is a studio smacked down, dead centre, in the middle of life . . . Against all the odds, and perhaps because the odds are against us, we make art.
>
> (Moon, 2002: 71)

The Community Table is influenced by the Portable Studio, a conceptual framework developed by Kalmanowitz and Lloyd (2005) to respond to contexts of conflict and upheaval. In it they emphasise the role of absorption and reference Wood when writing about art therapy studios: 'Human beings seem to have a basic need for absorption. Absorption is the opposite of alienation' (2000: 40).

The arts as crisis support

That the arts have a role to play at times of crisis has largely transcended country borders, politics, and cultures. Displacement is by its nature disorientating. The arts can support a place to pause, reminisce, remember, and recalibrate, as discussed in a World Health Organisation scoping report which synthesises the global evidence on the role of the arts in improving health and well-being throughout a person's life, in particular at times of crisis and distress (Fancourt & Finn, 2019).

The overarching aim of The Community Table model is to support people's resilience. It is informed by Psychological First Aid (PFA) (Lahad et al., 2013; WHO, 2011) and Siegel's idea of 'the window of tolerance' (2010), both focus on crisis intervention and support people to feel safe and grounded in the here and now. The authors have written elsewhere about working in a context of ongoing volatility and upheaval in northern France (Lloyd et al., 2018; Lloyd & Usiskin, 2020; Usiskin et al., 2020; Usiskin & Lloyd, 2020). Underpinned by trauma-informed practice, the work itself can act as a shelter for people existing in chaos, complexity, toxicity, and limbo, at times offering a means of protection and survival. These virtual shelters are made by what has often felt like an unconscious but collective desire to collaborate and create a space, on the part of both the art therapists and those taking part (Lloyd et al., 2018).

Art therapy, intersectionality, and social justice

It is necessary to apply an intersectional framework to all art therapy practice, not least when working with people who are displaced. 'Intersectionality is a way to understand how marginalized, intragroup identity differences simultaneously intersect to create and exacerbate experiences of oppression' (Kuri, 2017: 118). This author also suggests that art therapists need to understand how socially constructed knowledge and prejudice become internalised for both the therapist and those they work with, in spite of their skin colour or ethnicity. Kapitan states that art therapy, and the psychology it is based upon, has originated in the global North and West and been exported to different parts of the world, 'unconsciously replicating colonial patterns of cultural domination' (2011: 64). The Community Table has largely been visited by people from the global South and East (North Africa and the Middle East), many of whose countries have been occupied, colonised, or invaded at some point in history, distant and recent, by North European powers.

Talwar (2019) explores the intersection of art therapy, social change, and social justice in her edited book. This moves away from a focus on pathology towards 'models of caring' based on concepts of self-care, radical caring, hospitality, and restorative practice methodologies. Potash (2018) links art therapy with relational social justice. He further explores the idea of democracy: 'Looking more specifically at art therapy, it may be obvious how art promotes democracy by visualizing invisible injustices, providing a forum for representational voices, offering spaces to bring people together, and facilitating activities to imagine new solutions' (Potash, 2020: 3). Working with refugees in transit, injustices are played out on a daily basis through police violence and racial abuse, and Art Refuge, alongside the other organisations on the ground, has worked to offer a counter narrative. Through the sharing of images, narratives and context on social media, Art

Refuge aims to make the situation and human stories visible for a wider, public-facing audience (Usiskin et al., 2020).

Collaborative helping

Around The Community Table the Art Refuge team aims to be grounded in relational connection, as is both the attitude and the way in which the art therapists position themselves in response to others. Epston describes the commitment 'to meet people with compassion rather than suspicion' (1999: 140) while Madsen writes about collaborative helping which involves 'practices that help ground our work in a spirit of respect, connection, curiosity and hope' (2004: 1).

Community tables

The discipline of Art Therapy is culturally outside the frame of experience of most of those who have visited The Community Table in northern France, while the concept of community is familiar but often lost in displacement. The English language word 'community' derives from the Old French comuneté which comes from the Latin communitas, communis – shared in common (Oxford Dictionaries, 2021).

Community tables and meals are provided by charities and religious groups across the world within local communities: eating communally transcending cultures, countries, and religions. The artist Olafur Eliasson creates temporary communities around his immersive arts projects, often around tables, within which, as people encounter them, associations and memories are brought to the experience (Godfrey, 2019). Community lunches, festivals, and other social practices around tables have long been tools of socially engaged artists and participatory arts practices, going back to the 1970s. Conversation, relationships between individuals and communities, and social or political commentary often run alongside food (Singer, 2014).

Materials and media

Central to the work in northern France is considering what materials and media may link to culture and memory, and/or inspire and engage with people's imagination. The world has become more complex and so indeed has the visual language of artists. Moon questions whether 'a limited number of traditional fine art materials always provide an adequately complex visual grammar and syntax' (2010: 36). McNiff, writing in 1999, was already thinking about these ideas:

> I am always exploring what media do, how they affect us differently, what qualities they convey, how they influence the circulation of energy in spaces and in people, and how new media and new interactions among existing media improve practice.
>
> (1999: 197)

The authors propose that it is the responsibility of art therapists to look beyond traditional art materials and practices that might lack cultural relevance, particularly in contexts where there is need for social action and crisis intervention (Lloyd & Usiskin, 2020). Connection to a cultural continuum through access to world art history and contemporary arts practices helps give credence and value (Usiskin et al., 2020; Lloyd & Usiskin, 2020).

The specificity of materials and media used at The Community Table is thus a core feature of the work. Carefully sourced high-quality, pre-used materials offer a sense of history, gravitas, and culture being carried. For example, the building and rebuilding, made possible by the use of miniature bricks, can offer an imagined space, a zone between inner and outer reality. This material's tactility is significant and allows for play. Play provides an ability to lose oneself, become immersed, but it also allows for processing and reprocessing, moulding and reforming of a narrative (Lloyd et al., 2018) or a 'temporary home' (Dieterich-Hartwell & Koch, 2017: 1). These materials are offered alongside contemporary tools – mobile phones, video projectors, stop frame animation, and sound recorders.

The Community Table

From late summer 2015 Art Refuge worked inside tents, portacabins, and shipping containers in the large makeshift refugee camp (The Jungle). In October 2016 the camp was demolished and its population of 10,000 people dispersed. The Community Table model subsequently evolved to support the work in the dining room of a safe house, in a large open-plan community space, in a small apartment, and even online.

Refugee safe house

We were invited to work in the Maria Skobtsova safe house in late 2016. This small terraced house acted as temporary home and sanctuary for twenty or so vulnerable Eritrean and Ethiopian teenagers and young people, at any one time. Our team delivered an informal art making session around the dining room table for a few hours on Friday afternoons, before returning to the UK.

The remit of the house was to provide a safe space to support and sustain the necessary resilience that young people needed in coping with their situation. The house offered a welcoming 'family' environment in which individuals could rest and recuperate from physical and psychological experiences, as well as gain spiritual sustenance. Violence at the hands of the police in Calais had for many exacerbated vulnerabilities, making the local streets particularly precarious. The house became a necessary refuge.

While there were many poignant moments around the table, these were often disrupted. There might be unwanted news of a death or an injury or reports of the success of a high-risk journey to the UK. A new arrival might knock at the door asking for a change of clothes, shower, food, drink, or a place to sleep. On one occasion, we arrived to find the house full of sick teenagers as young as thirteen,

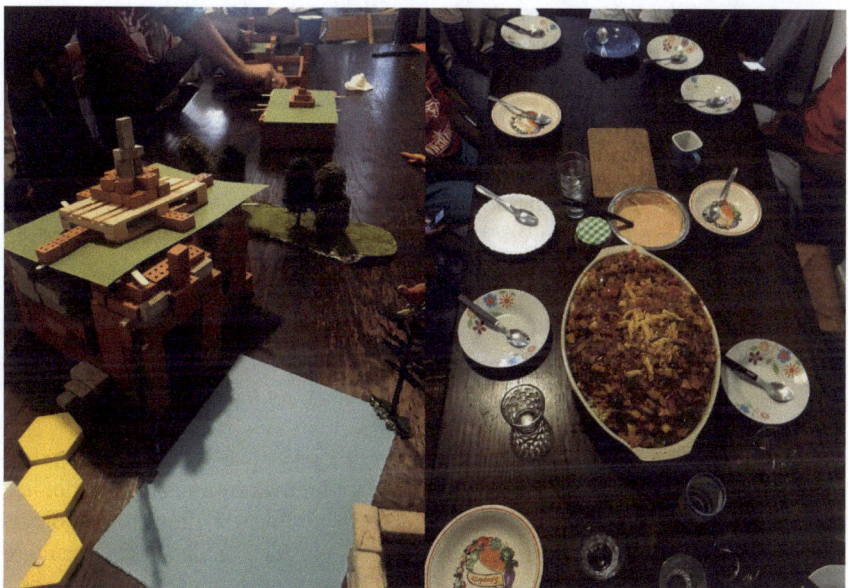

Figure 8.2 The dining room table in the safe house.

mostly upstairs in bed with flu and colds following the change to warmer, if wetter, weather. Clothes were drying on every surface including the backs of chairs around the table. Life in the house continued around us while a few young people gradually joined us at the table. Artworks were made, photographed or filmed, before the room was returned to its usual order to make ready for the evening meal.

On another occasion in September 2017 we sat around the dining table with a group of ten exhausted boys from Ethiopia and Eritrea, mostly visiting the house for showers and clothes washing, with one or two residents of the home among their numbers. Almost immediately, news of the death of a teenager known to members of the group brought those seated around the table to silence. The following extract is adapted from our fortnightly Facebook post written on the return journey back to the UK that evening.

> *Summer 2017*
>
> *The silence was gradually followed by a shift in mood as the young men began to tentatively build with the miniature bricks. One boy persevered with building a house with internal laid flooring and rooms, a sturdy roof, a terrace around the perimeter with trees and a Welcome sign over the entrance. He appeared to have created the safe house, and the other boys responded with admiration.*
>
> *In parallel, we were shown detailed journeys on mobile phones via Google Maps. These included the retelling of frightening events on route, such as*

being smuggled across the Sahara Desert and borders, and being held in prison in Libya. At the same time one of the boys explained that he had nothing left after his phone had been deliberately smashed by police. The night before he had jumped into the sea at the Calais port in an attempt to swim to the ferry, so desperate had he become to reach the UK. The other boys were worried about his safety.

The Eritrean youth worker, speaking in Tigrinya, clearly explained to the group why such risk taking behaviour needed to be countered with patience, emphasising that there were many people who cared about them all, both here and at home. The teenager responded by asking if he could borrow a mobile phone to speak to his mother back home in Eritrea.

We left the safe house in the knowledge that the early evening meal would take over the place of the art materials, food would be shared in a family-style gathering, before most of the boys headed back out into the evening.

We understood our role on a regular Friday afternoon as one in which we contributed to the ethos of the house, offering a space for art making and support, not just for the young people but for staff and volunteers who would often sit and join us together around the table. Over a period of years, we got to understand the culture and rhythms of the house, and each time we were reminded of the particular crisis context that underpinned it.

Refugee day centre

By contrast with the safe house, the day centre occupied a large warehouse space located near the port which could accommodate up to 350 people. The Community Table found its physical home in the form of a series of tables pushed together at one end of the room. The day centre also served as an informal meeting point for a number of organisations which would, like us, take over tables to deliver services such as English classes or send volunteers to sit and engage with the refugee population at different tables across the large room.

From the day the table was first set up in the large day centre in Calais, volunteers and humanitarian workers would sometimes join, appearing lost, even overwhelmed in the vast space. Initially, this left our team feeling conflicted, wondering if their presence at the table took resources away from the displaced population the centre was set up to serve. However, reflecting back to these early experiences, it was indeed the presence of staff, volunteers, and interpreters from across ethnicity, culture, religion, gender, generations, and socio-economic backgrounds that seemed to add to the richness of people's experiences.

The following extracts are taken from Facebook posts documenting three sessions and demonstrate how our work evolved in this particular setting.

September 2018
This week we brought a new material for the tabletop surface in the form of a large roll of black rubber flooring onto which we invited people to build

and draw. Two friends from Iran – a carpenter and an architect – were the first to join us, building together the Gate of all Nations from their hometown of Shiraz, before making other structures with the miniature bricks. The table attracted others from Sudan and Afghanistan. A PhD student from Japan also found his way to the table. The room filled with helpers and visitors and we realised that the day centre was starting to feel like a welcoming village hall with a sense of community, in spite of the increasing transience.

In May 2019, we decided to bring two manual typewriters to allow for a different sort of communication. We were also responding to the writing of a poem posted online by a refugee volunteer, marking another tragic death of a young Eritrean on the main Calais road the previous week. We wondered whether the typewriter might invite other verse.

May 2019

The daily preoccupation of avoiding the police violence and destruction of property carried on. Many already exhausted people were fasting in these conditions, while Ramadan was due to end in a few days time. The 1970s typewriters held a presence at the table and fitted with the other pre-used materials.

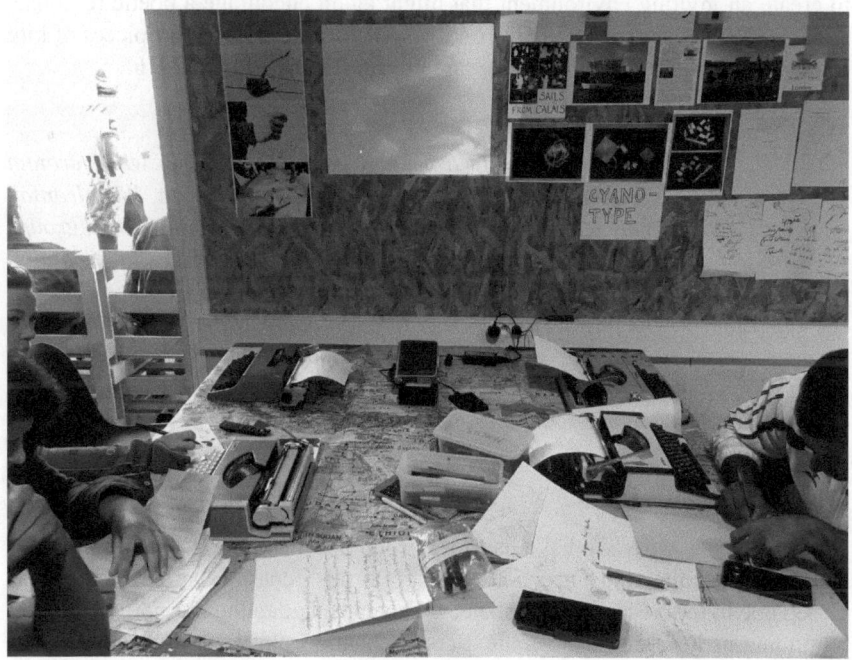

Figure 8.3 The Community Table in Calais.

In addition to a gentle stream of young men and a few women, there were a number of visitors in the day centre. These included a group of Italian nuns who were travelling across France, a first aid team and several volunteers from the other organisations who all came at some point to the table. Slowly, it found its rhythm and we were joined by a small group of Sudanese men who seemed particularly fascinated by the typewriters. Sitting alongside one of the nuns with whom he shared no common language was one young man from Sudan. Enamoured by the unusual 'machine', he managed to communicate some key autobiographical notes, typing over and over the name of his region, and at the same time trying to explain his local language.

The presence and use of the typewriters seemed to helpfully allow communication to be slowed down across languages, the pace of finding the correct keys perhaps also enabling some distance. The carbon paper, the idiosyncrasies of each machine, the mechanical keys, and in particular the sound of the tapping seemed to resonate, a cultural nostalgia gently stirred. A few men and a woman built with the bricks in amongst the typing, the sound of the keys seeming to offer a reassuring presence.

As with all our work, we chose materials and media in response to the emotional temperature in the room, alongside what we understood of the Calais context on that particular visit. A few months later we returned to some of the same tools. Laying out the typewriters, pens, and paper on the tablecloth map, we wanted to create an inviting environment that might again encourage a poetic response. Also, we created a projection area on the wall for a series of short pieces of kite footage taken during sessions in the large camp (The Jungle) in 2016.

September 2019
The films attracted curiosity from across the busy room, while around twenty people worked directly with us during the afternoon. With Iranian artist and team member Majid Adin leading the poetry writing, small groups of Farsi speakers gathered around the table. There was diversity of opinion and of language, with poems written and recorded in Farsi, Arabic, French and English. The interactions were at times intimate, with a mother and teenage son writing side by side, and others collaborating on poems. The kites, both flying high in the sky and caught in trees or on wires, offered a poignant metaphor for talking about the situation in Calais.

An apartment

At times in our work we have had to regroup and make new plans, as demonstrated in the following Facebook extract. On this occasion the day centre was closed due to unforeseen circumstances. This meant adapting our normal routine, reminding us how easily the context could change from week to week. The latter part of the afternoon was spent offering a smaller version of The Community

Table in an apartment in Calais, the cosy domain of someone who had recently gained asylum in France.

October 2017

We sat around the small table, sipping tea, us sitting with a group of men from Pakistan, Sudan, Afghanistan and Iran, chatting about the importance of equality for women, particularly with reference to education and driving. One of the friends reminisced about reading Jane Eyre in school, quoting parts of the book and discussing the characters and the Yorkshire Moor landscape that it was set in. Seemingly an unusual choice for an African schoolboy, he explained that the book was one of the reasons he wanted to come to the UK.

In this impromptu setting, we were guests in someone's home, 'smacked down' in the middle of life. The postcards mediated the space, their cultural range offering ways into conversation, encouraging metaphor, reminiscence, women's rights, politics, literature, and philosophy. The box of images was brought from the large day centre and acted as a bridge to our work and the culture we were starting to build in that other setting. This small group of men had variously sat at our table

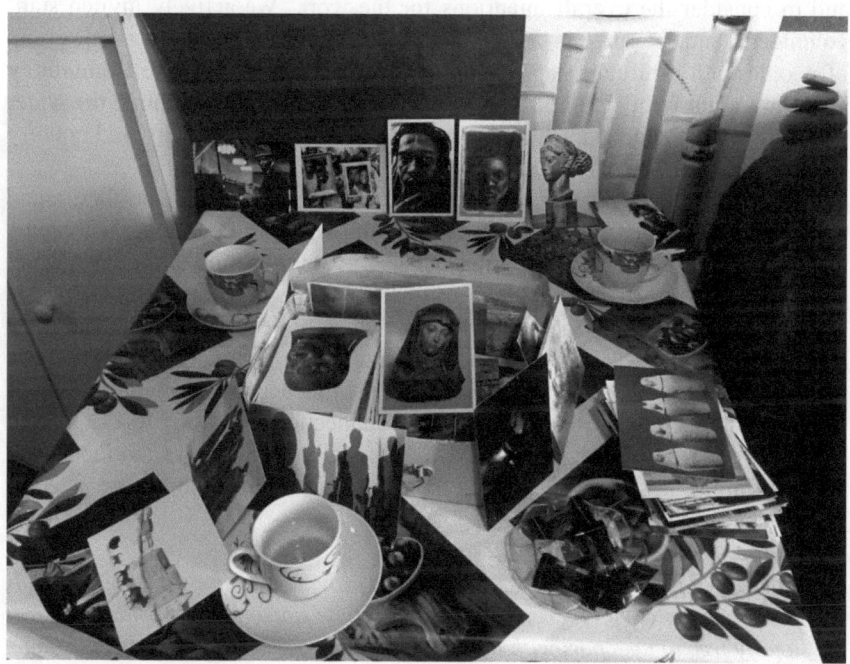

Figure 8.4 The apartment.

there. In this current intimate environment around a smaller version of The Community Table, we were the guests in someone's home. Here, we ourselves were treated with hospitality; there was a collaborative conversation in which complexities of race and gender in France, the UK, and in the men's own countries of origin were explored.

The Community Table Online and face-to-face in Paris

In mid-March 2020 we found ourselves unable to travel to France due to COVID-19. While the pandemic played out, the difficulties for refugees along the coast of northern France increased. This was due to heightened and unremitting police violence, intimidation, discrimination, and open displays of racism from police, far right groups, and individuals. It was exacerbated by the woefully inadequate COVID-19 response to refugees from the French state and the inevitable reduction in services from both French and British NGOs.

In response to the initial shock of the pandemic and the immediate need to adapt frontline services, we were invited to offer online training in Psychological First Aid for our French partner organisations. This made way for a further invitation to set up The Community Table Online to accommodate around fifteen people sitting at different tables on the videoconferencing platform of Zoom. We needed to once again adapt The Community Table to a new setting and to consider the overall intentions for the work. We actively invited staff, volunteers, and interpreters from our partner organisations and a small group of people with a refugee background who had taken part in The Community Table in Calais. While all sessions were co-facilitated by the authors, the wider Art Refuge freelance team was also able to join from across city and country borders, offering a network of support.

In a further development, we began to integrate online with on-the-ground delivery. The sessions ran in person at the Café Papote in Le Cedre, the Secours Catholique refugee day centre setting in Paris, at the invitation of the Paris team. We were subsequently invited to deliver three sessions of The Community Table Online and face-to-face, with the Art Refuge team projected onto a screen in the day centre as well as via laptops laid out on tables in an outdoor courtyard. We realised the potential for this new model in enabling access for a larger group of refugees without reliance on mobile phones, connection and data, while supported by the on-the-ground team. Hisham Aly, staff member at Secours Catholique who took part in the sessions, reflected on their importance in helping to create community spaces which had felt impossible before:

> In my own point of view, it's important to provide a centre working with vulnerable people with a creative and out of time space where participants feel totally free to take part with their own ideas and wishes. The impact is huge, not only socially but also there is a psychological aspect. The "I focus", "I exist" and "I express" factors greatly support a conversation even if we

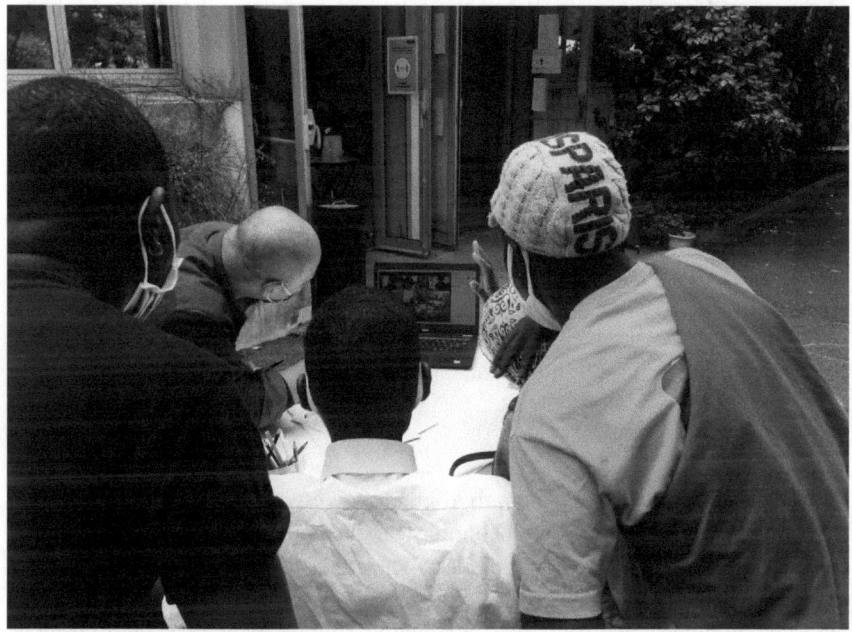

Figure 8.5 The Community Table Online and face-to-face. Photo credit: Secours Catholique – Caritas France.

don't speak the same language . . . that's how I saw this Community Table. By the way, we started talking about a community space.

(H. Aly, personal communication, October 8th 2020)

Discussion

In the examples described in this chapter, we actively adopted a responsive rather than reactive stance, ensuring the work was held professionally, responsibly, and confidently. Using the spirit of the art therapy studio, the parameters of Psychological First Aid and our commitment to the psychological safety of those participating, we needed to ensure careful boundaries around the work in this crisis context. This was not about exploring pathology but about shoring up resilience. We observed over time that there was the capacity for something convivial to happen around The Community Table, a shared interest and curiosity in others, shifting a little the idea of 'us and them'. Support could be mutual in the here and now. A cooperative, creative experience could take place, able to hold the multifaceted aspects of life at a specific point in time.

For each of the aforementioned examples, there have been necessary adaptations in response to context. In each setting, we have tried to understand the core principles that link back to the studio art therapy model and our stance as artists and art therapists. When we asked an asylum seeker from Afghanistan for feedback about The Community Table in the Calais day centre, he replied: "*The Community Table is like when you go to your grandmother's house, with an atmosphere like that, all people young and old; when I need time for myself, I go there*". His grandmother's house seemed to be a positive place for him that he saw as comfortable, intergenerational, and even a place where he could find time for himself. This response suggested how significant these points of meeting can be for people who have no family around them and may be looking for a sense of belonging. It also connected to our role as a group of mostly women working largely with groups of men, in which at times we have been addressed around the table as aunties, mothers, sisters, daughters, and even grandmothers.

Conclusion

Art Refuge has developed innovative, imaginative ways to work with refugees living in transit on the France–UK border who face ongoing exposure to hostility, cultural disorientation, and homelessness. The consistency of our presence in Calais over a five-year period has allowed for a culture to develop and a set of working tools, practices, and principles, adapted to context, which has manifested as The Community Table. This has emerged in response to a complex, changeable, and crisis context and as a way of defining the work, using the ongoing practice of assessment and formulation.

Out of this work we have developed an evolving model to be usable in wider contexts. We need to understand what this work might offer to each new setting, as each intermediary space has the potential to open up new possibilities for communication and connection. We know that online work can sometimes alienate. However, we have realised the need to persevere with exploring different permutations of The Community Table so that it can become a response to the bigger picture, the issues of our time, when more than ever we need to be gathering around real and imagined tables talking to each other, exchanging ideas, embodying the experiences, and seeking creative responses and solutions. This is not just for people who are like 'us' but between people from different genders, ages, ethnicities, cultures, ideologies, identities, socio-economic, and political backgrounds and from different perspectives.

All photographs: credit Art Refuge unless otherwise stated.

References

Anderson, H. (1997) *Conversation, Language and Possibilities*, New York: Basic Books.
Crane, R., Stanley, S., Rooney, M., Bartley, T., Cooper, L. & Mardula, J. (2014) 'Disciplined improvisation: Characteristics of inquiry in mindfulness-based teaching', www.

bangor.ac.uk/mindfulness/documents/DisciplinedImprovisation.pdf Accessed: September 14, 2020.

Dieterich-Hartwell, R. & Koch, S. (2017) 'Creative arts therapies as temporary home for refugees: Insights from literature and practice', *Behavioural Sciences*, 7:69, 1–11.

Epston, D.E. (1999) Co – research: The making of alternative knowledge. In: *Narrative Therapy and Community Work: A Conference Collection* (pp. 137–157), Adelaide, Australia: Dulwich Centre Publications.

Fancourt, D. & Finn, S. (2019) *What Is the Evidence on the Role of the Arts in Improving Health and Well-Being? A Scoping Review*, Copenhagen: WHO Regional Office for Europe; (Health Evidence Network (HEN) synthesis report 67).

Godfrey, M. (2019) *Olafur Eliasson, in Real Life*, London: Tate Publishing.

Kalmanowitz, D. & Lloyd, B. (eds.) (2005) *Art Therapy and Political Violence: With Art Without Illusion*, London and New York: Routledge.

Kapitan, L. (2008) 'Not art therapy: Revisiting the therapeutic studio in the narrative of the profession', *Art Therapy*, 25:1, 2–3.

Kapitan, L., Litell, M. & Torres, A. (2011) 'Creative art therapy in a community's participatory research and social transformation', *Art Therapy*, 28:2, 64–73.

Kuri, E. (2017) 'Toward an ethical application of intersectionality in art therapy', *Art Therapy*, 34:3, 118–122.

Lahad, M., Shacham, M. & Ayalon, O. (eds.) (2013) *The "BASIC Ph" Model of Coping and Resiliency: Theory, Research and Cross-cultural Application*, London; Philadelphia, PA: Jessica Kingsley Publishers.

Lloyd, B. & Usiskin, M. (2020) 'Reimagining an emergency space: Practice innovation within a frontline art therapy project on the France-UK border at Calais', *International Journal of Art Therapy*, 25:3, 132–142.

Lloyd, B., Usiskin, M. & Press, N. (2018) 'The Calais winds took our plans away: Art therapy as shelter', *Journal of Applied Arts & Health*, 9:2, 171–184.

Madsen, W. (2004) *Collaborative Therapy with Multi-Stressed Families*, 2nd edition, New York: Guildford Press.

McNiff, S. (1999) 'The virtual art therapy studio', *Art Therapy*, 16:4, 197–200.

Moon, C.H. (2002) *Studio Art Therapy: Cultivating the Artist Identity in the Art Therapist*, London: Jessica Kingsley.

Moon, C.H. (ed.) (2010) Introduction. In: *Materials & Media in Art Therapy: Critical Understandings of Diverse Artistic Vocabularies*, New York, Hove: Routledge.

Nolan, E. (2019) 'Opening art therapy thresholds: Mechanisms that influence change in the community art therapy studio', *Art Therapy*, 36:2, 77–85.

Oxford Dictionaries. (2021) https://www.lexico.com/definition/community. Accessed: December 8, 2021.

Potash, J. (2018) 'Relational social justice ethics for art therapists', *Art Therapy*, 35:4, 202–210.

Potash, J. (2020) 'We the art therapists: Democracy through creative action', *Art Therapy*, 37:1, 3–5.

Siegel, D. J. (2010) *'Mindsight', The New Science of Personal Transformation*, New York: Bantam Books.

Singer, F. (2014) 'Art and food: Better together?' Art Papers, www.artpapers.org/art-and-foodbetter-together/ Accessed September 18, 2020.

Talwar, S. (ed.) (2019) *Art Therapy for Social Justice: Radical Intersections*, London and New York: Routledge.

Usiskin, M. & Lloyd, B. (2020) 'Lifeline, frontline, online: Adapting art therapy for social engagement across borders', *International Journal of Art Therapy*, 25:4, 183–191.

Usiskin, M., Lloyd, B. & Press, N. (2020) 'Temporary, portable, virtual: Making galleries on the France-UK border at Calais'. In: *Art Therapy in Museums and Galleries: Reframing Practice*, edited by A. Coles & H. Jury (pp. 265–288), London: Jessica Kingsley.

Wood, C. (2000) 'The significance of studios', *Inscape: The Journal of the British Association of Art Therapists*, 5:2, 40–53.

World Health organization, War Trauma Foundation and World Vision International. (2011) *Psychological First Aid: Guide for Field Workers*, Geneva: WHO.

9 Transitioning into visibility

Exhibiting art from a therapeutic group for the intended purpose of knowledge sharing, education, social action, and social change in a northern Canadian community

Zoë Armstrong

This chapter explores how two art therapy groups were created, designed, and used for therapeutic purposes; and how the art that was created became a tool for change.

I live and work on the Traditional Territory of the Kwanlin Dün First Nation and the Ta'an Kwäch'än Council in Yukon Territory, which is home to fourteen First Nations with eight distinct languages. It is a land of diversity and extremes: the summer delivers twenty hours of daylight; the winter only about five. Summer temperatures can rise to 25°C and easily dip below -40°C in the winter. Yukon, the smallest of the three territories in Canada, is 482,443 km² and has a population of about 40,000 people, with 30,000 located in the capital of Whitehorse. The marginalised and invisible community that I work with on this land are transgender, Two-Spirit and/or nonbinary individuals. 'Two-Spirit' is a term used by First Nations peoples in North America in reference to gender identity (Armstrong, 2020). Myra Laramee is credited for coining this term in 1990 (Sylliboy, 2017) at the Annual International Gathering in Winnipeg.

Chase was my first client who identified as transgender. I met him when I was working at a not-for-profit organisation. He came into that first session surprised and a little confused when I introduced myself as the art therapist who would be working with him. He appeared slightly suspicious of the art therapy process but willingly shared that he was a trans man who was seeking support to cope with the impact of being fired from his job after being outed at work and discriminated against. Chase stated that he was not an artist and that he was not going to make any art as he did not believe that doing art would help him. Nevertheless, in that first session, he created his first piece of art and booked another session. This was the beginning of what became a safe, trusting, and long-standing therapeutic relationship and of my personal growth from ally to advocate.

About a year later, my business partner Erin Legault and I opened up our own private practice counselling agency. Because of my experience with Chase, I knew that, as cisgendered individuals, Erin and I needed more training to support the transgender, Two-Spirit and/or nonbinary community. We did our training with the

DOI: 10.4324/9781003095606-12

World Professional Association for Transgender Health (WPATH). We wanted our private practice to have a trans-informed lens, which included an understanding of the intersectional, overlapping, and interdependent systems of discrimination and disadvantage that individuals in this community may have been exposed to. We did not want any client that we worked with to have to spend time and energy educating us just to be able to access supportive services. We wanted to thoughtfully create a counselling space that was safe, welcoming, and inclusive for all clients.

Chase is a community leader who has a consulting business and founded All Genders Yukon to provide support to transgender, Two-Spirit, and/or nonbinary individuals, including the primary support people in their lives. Having appreciated how useful art therapy was for him to heal and express his emotions, Chase wanted to share with others what he had experienced. Two local nurse practitioners were facilitating a two-day workshop that they had organised on transgender health for the physicians at Whitehorse General Hospital and they asked me to present on art therapy. Chase attended the workshop to speak on his lived experience and was in the audience as I shared client–artist art and stories from my work with individuals who identified as transgender, Two-Spirit, and/or nonbinary, which were shared anonymously and with permission. Chase was there to witness the audience reactions to the art pieces created by himself and other people in the community that he did not know. Later, he told me how impactful the experience had been on two levels. The first level was impact of witnessing other individuals view the art that he and others had created, he felt seen and his experiences validated. The audience paid attention, you could hear and see their emotional reactions, which connected them to the All Genders community. This community was no longer invisible, abstract statistics turned into real stories of individuals with unique experiences and needs. Years later, I would overhear a doctor sharing with another doctor about the art that they saw at a conference being impactful and memorable. The second level was the power of seeing art made by other individuals from his shared community, seeing and understanding their experiences, the diversity and the similarity. For the first time he saw his authentic self and experiences reflected in other people. He stated that he no longer felt isolated and alone. Encouraged by the knowledge that Chase shared with me, and the impact the event had on him and the audience, I became committed to using art for knowledge sharing and educating others about the All-Genders community members with whom I worked.

Being invisible in a community occurs when an individual possesses multiple subordinate intersectional group identities, which is in contrast to those with a single subordinate group identity, who can be seen and have a sense of belonging within their group (Purdie-Vaughns & Eibach, 2008). Social invisibility results in being separated and systematically ignored by the majority of the public, leaving the individual feeling powerless. This was the experience of the transgender, Two-Spirit, and/or nonbinary individuals that I work with. Being invisible therefore results in being marginalised, as these individuals are pushed to and beyond the edges of a society (Dean, 2007).

Safe spaces for transgender, Two-Spirit, and nonbinary individuals are rare and needed for individuals to create community, build relationships, share information, and have their experiences be seen and witnessed. Providing art therapy groups emerged from this knowledge, an art therapy group could provide a place for this marginalised group to come together to create, share experiences, be witnessed by others, engage, and build community, while providing therapeutic care and information to resources. Chase, Erin, and I decided to create two groups; one group would be for individuals who identify as transgender, Two-Spirit, and/or nonbinary (All Genders), and a second group would be created for their significant others, friends, families, and allies/advocates (SOFFA). Funding needed to be secured to be able to offer this service, therefore my role as an art therapist expanded to include proposal and grant writing. In building on the knowledge that personalising and sharing the experiences of members of the All Genders community might improve our chances to secure funding, we adopted an unconventional approach. In addition to writing the proposal for funding, we asked for in-person meetings to share the art and stories of the individuals who would be benefitting from the funding. We were successful and able to offer weekly art therapy groups that alternated between the All Genders and SOFFA groups.

We wanted to create a welcoming art studio atmosphere where participants were free to decide how they participated. Groups ran for one and a half hours. To keep the confidentiality and safety of the individuals attending the groups they were held in the boardroom of our secure office. The back door of the building was available for anyone to enter or leave from and all bathrooms were gender neutral. Food was provided at each session, and there were always extras for people to take home, knowing that food scarcity was a daily worry for some of our participants. Sessions were held in the evening so that they did not interrupt standard work hours making them easier for people to attend. All ages were welcome, our youngest participants were six years of age and went all the way through to seniors. The groups were facilitated by Erin and I and up to twelve people could be seated around a large table, in the centre were art materials – oil pastels, markers, glue, scissors, paint, and clay. Holding the groups at our private practice gave us the option of using the individual counselling rooms if needed.

At the beginning of each session, confidentiality and safety were discussed and agreed upon. When everyone introduced themselves, they shared the pronouns they used. Sometimes individuals used this space to try out new names and pronouns. Individuals were encouraged to share what they needed from the group that day. Art directives were suggested, and we would share the agenda for the group, for the first half there would be art making and for the second half of the group we would share art and have discussion. At this point, we would stress that participation may look different for everyone at the group. For some individuals attending the group was enough for them, for others it may be making art. Everyone was invited to share the art that they made, but it was not mandatory to do so. If someone decided to share their art, they would be asked if they just wanted to share it, say something about it, or be comfortable enough for others to comment and discuss it with them.

During art therapy groups, individuals shared their lived experience, shared knowledge, and built a network of resources. While they were making art, conversations were more light-hearted. Information was shared on where a safe place was to get a haircut, what medical doctor was supportive, what their day was like, or a success that they wanted to celebrate. It also became a place where individuals donated clothes to others who needed clothes to be able to present themselves more authentically, the bathrooms became changing rooms.

When it came time for the participants to share their art, there was a noticeable shift in the discussions, and they switched from light-hearted to a much deeper, more vulnerable place. They shared the difficulties of fertility treatments, medical transitions, and social transitions. The impact of discrimination, microaggressions, being misgendered, and consequences of being outed, or authentically presenting themselves, lack of housing, struggles with employment, loss and grief of histories, families, friends, and missed opportunities were discussed. Dealing with administration and how to change identification documents was shared. What came through all of these discussions was the lack of informed services, lack of safe spaces, and the discrimination they faced while trying to get their needs met. Members shared deep feelings of frustration and desperation, they wanted to raise awareness of their needs. They wanted the opportunity to access support and resources from informed, educated, competent, and compassionate transgender healthcare providers and changes in public policy.

The creative process and the created art image are powerful carriers of meaning that can be harnessed and exhibited before diverse audiences (Leavy, 2020). With this understanding, I suggested to the All Genders and SOFFA groups the idea of a public art exhibition of the work that they had created in group art therapy. The client-artists embraced this idea. They wanted to be seen and to have agency, to have a voice in their community by sharing their art and personal stories in a safe, anonymous way that minimised fear and consequences to sharing. The group took ownership of how they wanted to present themselves by deciding and directing how they wanted to do it.

The group's decision to curate and exhibit art in a gallery or public exhibition space was only the beginning. As their art therapist, my role now included writing a proposal to a local art gallery, Arts Underground, which held juried exhibitions. When the proposal was successful, and the art gallery agreed to host the art exhibition, the client-artists reviewed all of the art that they had created in their art therapy groups and selected the pieces they wanted to display. The gallery required at least 70% of the art on display to be for sale. It was decided that each piece would be priced at the cost of a single therapeutic session. This price would demonstrate the financial resources that are needed to receive mental health support. In addition, the client-artists had to write an artist statement to go with each piece, putting into words the inspirations, motivations, and stories associated with their artworks. They chose the titles of their piece, whether to remain anonymous or create a pseudonym, how they wanted to describe their gender identity, and what pronouns they use.

John Dewey (2005) believed that art was a compelling means by which a community can be strengthened and mobilised for political action. To publicise the show, the art gallery produced posters and postcards that were distributed around Whitehorse, and it was announced in the events section of the newspapers.

Artist statement for Figure 9.1: 'There are many trans individuals who suffer like I do. We need more resources and for you to understand and support us'.

Figure 9.1 Poster for the art exhibition Transitioning Into Visibility. Original art: *It's a Horrible Wonderful Trans Life* (18" x 24") by Nikolas Caelan Glaeser (gender identity: male; pronouns: he/him or they/them).

The art therapy groups considered who their audience should be and whom in particular they wanted to attract and for what purposes, then individual invitations to the show were emailed directly to them. On the opening night, a 'soft' private opening occurred an hour before the public opening so that anyone who was concerned about possible consequences or discrimination or was not able to be open about their gender in public for various reasons could view the show safely before the general public arrived. Client-artists who chose to share their art publicly found that this was a safe way to engage their families, friends, and the larger community to be involved in their healing process and raise public awareness. It was critically important to be thoughtful about who should be invited to attend the art exhibition and why. Policymakers were among the people strategically targeted by the client-artists to be invited to view the art exhibit as part of an explicit goal of social change. Teachers and their classes were invited with education as the primary goal. Journalists were invited to promote the art exhibition to the public, so as to gain a broader viewing audience and educate the public. One important function of the art exhibition was to increase understanding and possibly find commonalities between viewers and the client-artists, which can begin to happen only when individuals who belong to this invisible and marginalised community are no longer invisible.

The painting Chase chose to exhibit depicted the first time he considered killing himself in a public and shocking way. His idea developed from deep feelings of frustration and desperation to raise awareness of the needs of individuals who are transgender, Two-Spirit, and/or nonbinary. Specifically, he needed an opportunity to access support and resources from informed, educated, competent, and compassionate transgender healthcare providers and for supportive public policy. Chase did not want to die, but he felt he was out of options to secure the supports needed for him and his invisible, marginalised community.

Artist statement for Figure 9.2: 'This piece is about the first time I considered killing myself in a public way out of desperation to get YG [Yukon government] to help us. There is a faceless politician on the bridge, the politicians have ignored us for years. They know how much help we need but make excuses. Perhaps if I hung myself from the Riverdale bridge, or drove into the legislative with a note . . . maybe, just maybe they would help our community. We have tried everything and there are no options left. The words are in NDP orange because they are the only ones who have helped, but they don't have the seats to truly help us'.

Contemporary gallery exhibition spaces have evolved their mission of educating the public beyond passive learning and the display of art to interactive engagement that can foster personal growth and community awareness of societal needs (Peacock, 2012; Treadon et al., 2006). We provided a small space for exhibit attendees to engage in art making and asked them to leave their art so that it could be an anonymous exchange between them and exhibiting client-artists, to let them know that they had been seen and heard. After the art exhibition had closed, I brought all of the art that had been created by exhibit attendees to the groups and hung it on the walls for them to see, to concretely know that they had been seen, heard, and responded to.

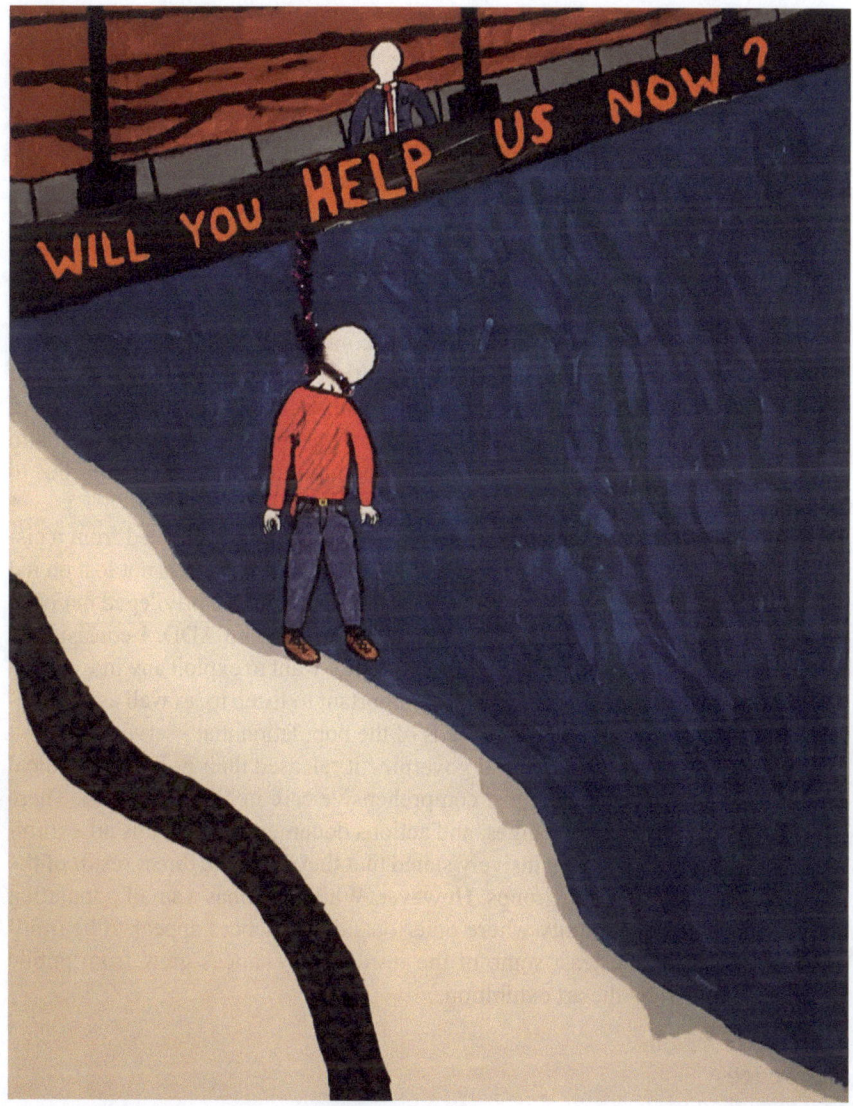

Figure 9.2 The Politician (18" x 24") by Chase (Identity: trans/transmasculine; pronouns: he/him).

The art exhibition, *Transitioning Into Visibility*, consisted of thirty pieces of art. Each piece of art was framed and hung with respect and dignity. It was held for the month of May in 2018 and 4,320 individuals, representing 15% of the population of Whitehorse, visited the art exhibition. The art exhibition was initially intended to be displayed for the month of May but was extended until the end of June at the request of the art gallery. Five pieces of art were sold on the opening night, and eight pieces of art were sold in total. Informing client-artists that their art had been sold produced a variety of emotions. Surprise was consistently expressed by all eight people; no one was expecting to sell their art. They said that it brought a smile to their face and increased their feeling of self-worth and confidence. Not only were they seen but also valued, and people prove this by buying their art. Client-artists shared that the money they earned from the sale went to buy food and basic necessities.

The awareness created by the art exhibition helped in providing additional funding to both continue art therapy groups and for mental health supports for the All Genders community. Art therapy groups using an art-focused studio approach provided the opportunity for individuals to continue to build community and confidence. Without this, creating an art exhibition for the intentional purpose of sharing knowledge, education, social action, and social change would not have occurred. The purpose of the art therapy groups was not to learn coping skills to exist within the oppressed and marginalised community that they live in but to create change in the culture of Yukon Territory.

Notably, most of the research on gender thus far has been conducted from a cis-gender, heteronormative, androcentric, and gender binary view. It is not lost on me that I am white, cisgender, straight, and live as a member of the privileged majority in my community even though I struggle with dyslexia and ADD. I consistently and robustly examine my implicit biases and do not want to exploit any individuals with whom I work. For these reasons, it is important to listen to, as well as collaborate with, the thoughts, wishes, and needs of the population that I serve.

In March 2021, Yukon Territorial government released their policy on medical transgender care, and it is the most comprehensive care in North America. There were many social impacts, changes, and actions documented since this art exhibition, though none can be conclusively stated that they were the direct result of the art exhibition or art therapy groups. However, Whitehorse has a small population that is an isolated community where other outside influences appear to be minimal, suggesting that at least some of the results and changes grew from public awareness created by the art exhibition.

References

Armstrong, Z. (2020). *Transitioning Into Visibility: A Longitudinal, Retrospective Study Tracing the Social Impacts of Exhibiting Therapeutic Art Created by Transgender, Two-Spirit, and Nonbinary Individuals*. Doctoral dissertation, Mount Mary University.

Dean, H. (2007). Marginalization, Outsiders. In *The Blackwell Encyclopedia of Sociology*. American Cancer Society.

Dewey, J. (2005). *Art as Experience*. London, Penguin.

Leavy, P. (2020). *Method Meets Art: Arts-Based Research Practice* (3rd ed.). New York, Guilford Publications.

Peacock, K. (2012). Museum Education and Art Therapy: Exploring an Innovative Partnership. *Art Therapy, 29*(3), 133–137.

Purdie-Vaughns, V. & Eibach, R. P. (2008). Intersectional Invisibility: The Distinctive Advantages and Disadvantages of Multiple Subordinate-Group Identities. *Sex Roles*, *59*(5), 377–391.

Sylliboy, J. R. (2017). *Two-Spirits: Conceptualization in a L'nuwey Worldview*. MA thesis, Mount Saint Vincent University. http://ec.msvu.ca:8080/xmlui/bitstream/handle/10587/1857/JohnRSylliboyMAEDThesis2018%20%28Master%20of%20Arts%20in%20Education%29.pdf.

Treadon, C. B., Rosal, M., & Wylder, V. D. T. (2006). Opening the Doors of Art Museums for Therapeutic Processes. *The Arts in Psychotherapy*, *33*(4), 288–301.

10 The wall inside

Painting with young offenders

Ben Wakeling

Core to the project is that patients use art as an expressive tool, and draw from imagination. Centring the patients' experiences, emotions, and memories, the project gives patients a tool to aid self-reflection and transformation of difficult emotions.

(McGrath et al., 2019: 30)

Introduction

The expressive graffiti and well-being arts programme is a weekly programme for service users from Barnet Enfield and Haringey Mental Health Trust (BEHMHT), across the whole life span, which seeks to sustain people's recovery from mental health difficulties, enable them to believe that they can start to get their lives back on track and be part of their community, as well as reinforcing a positive sense of well-being. This project crosses the service lines of BEHMHT – child, youth, adult, and elder – as well as involving the Outsider Gallery and the University of East London (UEL).

An inpatient art studio needs to be a responsive and flexible space and is particularly necessary because they are working not only with creativity but also with people who are having diverse and dynamic experiences of distress and madness. Creating a responsive space also means trying to put the person first, centring their needs and desires from the first session onwards. Part of the power of creative practice is to allow people to both explore and explode their sense of self. In terms of exploration, generating self-awareness is a powerful and scary moment to be in, but if achieved can help to turn things around for an individual.

Outsider Gallery's art programme at BEHMHT North London Forensic Service has been running since 2016. For each intervention all eleven wards are considered, then with one chosen four to six patients are referred to the twelve-week programme. One of the programme's most efficient tools is to react to service users. Over ten weeks (contact time) service users will be offered individual sessions as well as working within a group setting. The art programme occupies a studio space that progresses through to using the Therapy Wall. If given permission, I will document the programme with a 35mm film camera. Outside of this

DOI: 10.4324/9781003095606-13

programme, photographs as well as the original outcomes or artwork can be hung and exhibited at the Outsider Gallery if there's acceptance from all involved and most importantly, it is what's best for the person. In these opportunities with the gallery, patient welfare is our first and only priority.

With the extension into the gallery, the art programme also seeks to promote a culture of peer support through the creative activity with opportunities for performance (exhibitions) that will be reinforcing of their recovery and also empower some of the service users to feel able to contribute to a wider community network. Outsider Gallery has the potential structure to deliver public events that will involve community and voluntary sector organisations from across the community. This helps people feel able to connect and belong, as well as challenge some of the stigma and misunderstanding about mental health that happens within institutions as well as in the general community.

Central to the art programme is the Therapy Wall – a large, paintable, outdoor wall surface that a service user is invited to paint on. The service user is informed that the wall will be whitewashed after every session. This is for two reasons. First, as it's in communal areas of a secure unit, whitewashing ensures a level of privacy and confidentiality for service users with an aim at building trust. The second reason protects the first; knowing that it can be whitewashed can often help release possible tension and allow painting with a more frantic honesty, an approach that can excite and encourage – as most of us are discouraged from an early age of drawing on the wall.

I believe expressions need to be met with cautious observation; this is after all a clinical, medically led environment and rightly so. Encouraging and allowing room for expressions is considered radical. This programme seeks to impact on both the individual and the institution itself. On the individual, this work seeks to help people better understand themselves, develop their self-confidence, their self-belief, sustain their recovery, and promote their overall well-being. The impact on the service is conveyed in this statement by Dr Katrin Edelman, Clinical Director Haringey:

> Part of the power of this type of creative work is the impact that it can have on the relationship between the staff and the client group. Care coordinators are often amazed at seeing how well their clients can engage in creative media and performance, as their regular encounter with the client is to see someone more defined by the deficits of their psychopathology rather than their strengths and assets – what makes them manage and cope on the day to day. This shift of perspective of the client is part of what is needed for an embedding of the Enablement approach across the Trust.
>
> (Personal communication, 2016)

Observing and beginning

At the beginning of the twelve-week programme, I sit down and discuss the ward staffs' observations. From these early conversations between us to when the programme, or more specifically, the contact time begins, varies as situations for service users can change quickly. Patients get moved or transferred, observations shift, solitary confinement is a problem, and relationships in every possible capacity will continue to evolve and behavioural moods affect their own actions and developments.

Past information and the long-term past behaviour about a service user can, however, be too much for me; having that knowledge too early on disrupts my opportunity for seeing a person with a first impression. Approaching our relationship with openness can, I believe, have a profound impact on how our relationship(s) with a service user develops. A forensic hospital sits both in between and with the mental health psychiatric service and the justice system, where problems and expressions linked to hierarchy and authority may be defused. The Therapy Wall approach has the potential to put me in a more equal position to connect where I can expose staff to a service user's attributes rather than working within the hierarchy of the system, allowing me to manoeuvre around those systemic barriers. That knowledge – of data and case history – can come later in our relationship and for me it can come to light when engaging in the Therapy Wall. It allows more honesty for all those involved, more responsibility to share, express, and build trust. This step needs constant care and attention as breaking away from hierarchy-led programmes without due consideration can cause risk.

Disruption from service users and troubled wards can be a starting point for us. All staff are vital to the art programme and its framework. Discussions with Occupational Therapy (OT) staff and clinicians enables further understanding of my approach and presents a space in which I too can reflect on the work. This acts as a bridge for my introduction to the ward. Listening to staff's reflective thoughts of individuals' current mood state and conditions (behaviours) over the past week and previous hours are very important, as well as citing all noteworthy happenstances. Also, clinicians and psychologists will be informed at some point from other internal discussions with staff and perhaps service users, of our programmes as we all begin to link in with each other's workings.

The working relationships with the occupational therapists has been a revelation for me. Having a trusted, hard-working confidante has helped maintain my focus and drive throughout each clinic. Unfortunately, these close working relationships can be short-lived as all wards are contained separately, so by default staff are assigned to each of the wards respectively. In reflective moments like this I can't help but acknowledge all the wonderful, empathetic hard work from individuals in this job role.

There's almost a saved amount of energy, which helps redistribute a creative freedom when being able to work with staff members who are able to be open and non-judgemental, thus allowing vital moments of expressive direction without causing friction between the facilitators and the service user(s). It all needs to be constantly maintained, simply because more people in a room creates more dialogue and possible distractions. I want to alleviate possible distractions and foster the desire for self-awareness. I want to feel able to creatively roam when working alongside staff, and OTs have that quality. They are psychically with me and with no friction I can direct, and we collaborate.

Before I meet new referrals, there's now a considered thought in place whereby the OT working on that ward would mention the project very briefly in perhaps a service user and staff meeting or on ward rounds or even just in passing. There are very gentle nudges in this programme. At a later date I arrange a time to come in and spend the afternoon on the ward. These mini stages are taken into account because it can be easy to overwhelm someone. I'm not positioned as a therapist, this isn't occupational therapy, the wall isn't a mural. So I begin in the communal areas, the open communal living room is a good place to navigate around, it has sky television, comfy sofas, and it's where I'll place myself to interact. Being that I'm a new face, I'll get questions. Entertaining ones, personal, inappropriate ones, some are interested, and there's an inquisitive nature in the air. I find these moments special, and they are common, it's normal human behaviour that I can empathise with, but it's also very complicated to interact with.

Ideas may be lacking when you're asking someone to come out of their shell a little and be creative, but life stories are theirs and often where I try to begin. It's where I can learn about their individual needs. These moments don't have a one-size-fits-all attitude either but rather, intuitive behaviours that are listened to – that's my high-profile risk and a strategy that institutions don't often allow. That first meeting with the service user(s) is very important, some of my details of the programme itself can be vague but that can help stimulate engagement. The idea of drawing on a wall with spray paint can excite so that is usually mentioned, but trust in the relationship isn't there yet and I'm continually considered as an outsider.

Although unconventional, I do reveal some information about myself. It's limited and centred around art life but it's useful; remembering that this is an experimental expressive arts programme in a forensics unit and my ideas to service users are new. For some, this first meeting can be a really exciting moment. The communal area is a neutral position, it's an environment where I'm not giving instructions, the hierarchy is much more even at this stage and by not instigating anything, there's room for equality in the conversation. Conversations can include politics, art and music, cultures, religious views, current affairs, and ideas. A lot of service users are preoccupied by profound philosophical issues and centring these conversations and actions around art as a way to express them can be a lot easier for some.

Early sessions of group and 1–1 interventions

I am on an all-male ward in a forensic mental health unit. The environment is tight, fragile, and clinical. In such environments, a group will only be able to occur if there's some degree of tolerance between the service users prior to the programme. The setting is usually a small multipurpose room for varied consultations in all capacities, therapies, etc., but for me it's my art studio – to my best ability – as I can't change a thing in there! In the room are a few heavy chairs, a table on wheels, and a window that hardly opens, old used magazines, and maybe an exercise or entertainment object – not ideal for a painter's art studio, but you have to make the best of it and be as resourceful as you can.

With both group and 1–1, I usually start with a big piece of canvas and this canvas I treat as my gateway. More often than not I want to awaken those feelings of rebelliousness in that room when I begin describing what the possibilities are. Except for some house rules, people like hearing that there's no rules, that we will allow what might be. The instructions are simple, spontaneity is encouraged . . . and it has been known, at times, that I would also encourage drawing and painting on any part of that room.

In this first contact session, service users and myself will draw together, this huge canvas that we can paint on will see us taking it in turns to quickly make a mark, write/use words, to respond without thinking for too long. So I'll encourage impulsiveness if necessary, we'll stand up if possible as I believe this can get us into that excitable energy. I try to translate this into expressive roaming and creating a visual language. This will hold and allow the trauma to be present. Barrages of paint will happen and naive marks beginning to occur, there's that energy in the room I mentioned, and it needs to be used – so encouragement keeps being applied. It's quick, vocal, and comments along with references will often come out from the service user(s). Comments range from what is currently being drawn to verbal disruption. I will certainly be asked questions as I'm a new face on the ward and yes I do respond, and I show caution and respect with it – I have to. But at the same time, I do and I don't block that direction of traffic, which again some may say this helps break down barriers, hierarchy can be seen as dismantled within this programme, but in truth what occurs is a trusting relationship that has respect and shows a willingness to engage. Keeping my instructions and questions simple and clear we can often (at some point in the session) discuss what they have come out with. I sometimes like to imagine a sense of being in the trenches together, a solidarity of emotions perhaps, I often feel that connection and it has the power to be felt and so someone would usually talk and explain what's been drawn. The reason why they have drawn something can be brought up as well, or thoughts of an ideology and a fictional story may have been created by taking it in turns to respond to each other's marks on the large canvas in front of us.

The second session mirrors the first. I'll introduce the sketch book. It'll be brand new, unwrapped, and offered to anyone attending the second appointment. As the inside joke goes 'I'll bribe 'em with tea and biscuits' – the sketch book is my tea and biscuits. Again some options are put to the group, simple interactions between us and I don't say much. As they unwrap the book last week's work is underneath, rolled out across the big table. This will be the first time they have seen the works or outpouring created during last week's session and so this is all happening at the same time. If I were to speak, potential inspiration and ideas could be missed, so I simply wait and observe.

Attempting to put this environment together each week can be exhausting and can make me feel anxious because the room does have to be put together. It's a multipurpose room, so it's clinical and blank but for what's now beginning to be understood about this programme – more of a professional art studio is needed.

Therapy Wall

This quote from a theoretical paper about our Graffiti and Wellbeing Programme sets the scene:

> Unlike many street art projects in health or secure environments the graffiti wall in this project was not an end product, but a continuous and ongoing process. There was no final mural being worked towards, which would then exist in a static state. The project thus remained true to the processual and ephemeral nature of graffiti art practice, which can always be erased, written over, or in other ways altered by official or unofficial means. The fact that the wall was always in process rather than becoming a final object can also be seen as an effective tactic to keep the institution at bay. A mural requires permissions, sign off, risk assessment, including, presumably, approval of the 'final image' for inclusion in the unit. By keeping the wall in process, these permissions were sidestepped, enabling the expression of the usually disallowed.
>
> (McGrath et al., 2021: 19)

Crime, art, and mental health. The wall sits in a space that can harness and create an expressive language for the most vulnerable and also at the same time provide a viewing platform for staff perspectives and views – to shift! Nothing is off limits of what you can write and paint. After every session the wall is documented photographically and painted over. Every client is able to keep a copy of every wall that they have painted, which they receive in the closing sessions.

Drawing on a wall – historically and currently policed by all types of authority personnel – is another reason this programme keeps its edge and can feel like an unauthorised act. Because the whole wall is erased after every session it can often create a spark of being truthful and it's with this shift within the service user that enables the wall to ignite self-awareness – an integral part of the road to maintaining recovery. Being able to use an exciting medium, and engage in an act that normally incurs trouble, has produced incredible results in the context of the recovery model.

This creative, expressive arts programme also has the potential to be very exploratory and some staff feel the wall to be potentially dangerous. It can become explosive when emotions, tensions, and personal stories come to the front. That expression is not often encouraged in this hypersensitive environment, but when it does emerge complete attention is needed by staff to keep everyone safe.

Painting over the wall has sometimes proved tricky, when brilliant moments of clarity and honesty have appeared in a visual format, the act of painting over so soon after its creation has led to deflated confidence, but by keeping the photograph moments can be remembered. This is where the camera and the art of photography becomes an integral part of the wall. A smartphone would be easier but feels tacky given its links to social media – plus smartphones and similar technology are not allowed in this environment. The 35mm camera feels more professional. The promise that I will process the film and they can have copies of everything helps ease the goodbye of the work, allows the patient to remind themselves months and perhaps years later what they did in that moment where they were seen, where hierarchy was dismantled, and expressive honesty was given a safe foundation to erupt on.

Finishing the programme at the wall often feels inappropriate and the majority of the time there's an agreement to have our last session back in the art room. If we are lucky, there's a cup of tea and biscuits to accompany us as we sit together and talk.

Conclusion

Away from the wall and the session itself can lie a range of staff opinions. This work is often referred to as a graffiti project. I personally understand the values of traditional graffiti – and this project isn't 'graffiti' but sure has its roots there and it certainly isn't street art either – a distinct difference is one acts without permission entirely and the other is a monetised, legal version of the former. This programme however could be considered in a constant transition. As noted earlier, the Therapy Wall can also sidestep many permissions that would be needed for a mural for example. What's become interesting is that the early stages of using the wall provide space for the anger and aggression – the negative response – to come out and often a person will eventually start drawing or painting something else. I think that is a very special tool to give them because after the anger, the negative can hopefully give way to something else.

Before interest in my accidental approach led to a commissioned art programme in forensics, there was a time when painting walls in unfamiliar territory without permission was a compulsive necessity for me. In truth, it still is. Being told not to paint is familiar to me, by institutions, even at school, unless it's done in a manner that authority deems appropriate; I've been discouraged throughout my life from painting, but visually expressing myself through dark complex thoughts saved my life. These experiences inform and mould the Therapy Wall approach.

References

McGrath, L., Ayorendi, O., Biskin, B., Liebert, R.J., Kilday, S., & Mighetto, I. (2019). *Graffiti Art and Wellbeing Project Service Evaluation*. UEL Clinical and Community Evaluation Team.

McGrath, L., Mighetto, I., Liebert, R., & Wakeling, B. (2021). Stuck in separation: Liminality, graffiti arts and the forensic institution as a failed rite of passage. *Sociology of Health and Illness*, Online First.

11 Inside–outside

On being art focused

Steve Pratt

This chapter is about my work as an art psychotherapist with emphasis on being 'art focussed' as the primary mode of engagement. I discuss my ways of working, which tested the boundaries of how I learnt to do art therapy with people who require physical as well as mental containment, where the only way of engaging was to create the concrete boundaries of a safe container to make art. Amongst the work, I also present fragments from my own background that provide insight into how, in this demanding work, we are constantly forced back on ourselves to re-examine the fragile resources we carry in order to endure some of the most murderous counter transference feelings whilst always returning to concentrate on the art object as the only way of maintaining sanity.

Fragment 1

SESSION 15

I'm carrying an Assault ladder towards the fuselage of a Boeing 737, a long time in the past. We are about to jettison the doors from the outside and assault into the rear of the aircraft to rescue the hostages. I'm in the front. We repeat these actions every day for the time I'm on the Counter Terrorist team. The experience is ingrained into my responses. That's how traumatic memory works; seemingly unrelated experiences get trapped, waiting for release into the everyday possibility for catastrophe. It could be a smell, a sound, or a feeling in the body. It's a fragment I'm unaware of, as I carry the easel into the observation room on the segregation unit. It must be something to do with the awkward nature of the easel and the need for silence because if I make a noise the client will wake up, and it'll cause all hell to break loose. In the process of leaning the easel, I catch my foot on a chair and the whole thing clatters to the floor. The doors explode outwards, and we slither through the gap. The client is now up, screaming at the window in front of me, headbutting the window harder and harder. I bring in the explosive charges of art materials. This will calm things down.

DOI: 10.4324/9781003095606-14

The therapist

I came to art therapy after almost thirty years of making art myself, following on from a seventeen-year military career. I found art helped 'to make sense of things'. Not as a verbalised narrative to give meaning to the pieces I made but as a way of transforming experience through (doing) non-verbally. It was impossible to talk about the pieces I made – they just made sense through the act of making.

The client

This account of art therapy covers a period where events have moved on. The client is no longer in the terrible space I describe. In fact, it could be that they were never present. It's a snapshot of an experience from a particular perspective. The impression that came to mind when I was first introduced was 'forlorn'. He has been on hunger strike for some time and does not wash. Staff are often assaulted, particularly during nasal gastric feeding. Violent outbursts are a way of protecting himself. Self-harm in the form of head banging and self-punching partially negates the terrible thoughts that invade his mind.

The setting

The client is attended to by a dedicated team. Like them, I volunteered for the work. In the army, they say 'never volunteer'. My sessions with this client are for twenty minutes daily. There are other units that I visit in the institution, but none of the people I see talk about their work. Art is our point of contact. Art enables me to be inside and outside the arrangements that brought me here – I think of myself as artist in residence, in the hope that I can gain a creative perspective to the work, but mostly I feel a sense of paralysis, of being unable to process any kind of creative thought.

Fragment 2

SESSION 50

It's my turn on watch, staring blindly through a starlight scope into the dark with my rifle at the ready. Night after night for three months at a time – for longer than was healthy. There was talk of throats being cut. Appears (suddenly) like a pale apparition at the three-quarter length observation window; like the shock of seeing one's own shadow come to life. When he turns away I glance a look at the way he moves; athletic, capable, striding purposefully for three strides, shoeless with odd socks, momentarily comical but frightening too – to the windowsill for the jumble of papers, drawings, scraps of paper, paper cups, tissues, scattered here and there. Returns, bends down and pushes a piece of paper under the door. It's a drawing of a country house with garden and fence, cleverly drawn, which I later find impossible to reproduce due to the weight and confidence of each pencil mark. All his drawings were made in private. Over the days other drawings follow; a fox and a rabbit that were given names, a horse, a cow, and some sheep in landscape settings. This was the productive period. Then the drawings stop.

Aim, method, and content

The aim, established through clinical supervision, is to provide a safe and consistent work container by adapting the structured open studio (see Bonneau, 2017) that I was using. We are separated by a partition door with a half-length plate glass window. There is an observation area where the duty staff can monitor his every move on CCTV. Verbal communications are possible, but the client resorts to hand, face, and body gestures, with occasional handwritten messages held up to the window. My medium of communicating is by drawing and painting.

The client is highly sensitive to visual material; he fearfully refuses picture content generated from books or TV and no picture material is accepted into his space. At the suggestion of presenting a colouring book or a photocopy he moves away fearfully, but drawings generated by my own hand are accepted and viewed closely – as if being judged. Expressive content is denigrated; a circulating single finger pointing to the head suggests the art therapist is not quite right in the head. This brings a smile to my lips, and I wonder if, by a nod of the head, I'm undermining my very own existence. Pictures of figures relating are usually met with fearfully generated violent self-destructive responses or with derogatory gestures. Safety for the client lay in nature scenes – horses, hens, dogs, birds, in a fantasy farm, or forest landscape. Scenes adapted from 'Colouring Book 1' are drawn out and painted to near completion by myself before being taken into the space on an easel for completion through interactive engagement with the client. Preparation time is at least sixty minutes. Three colour palettes with a full range of colours for the client to point and choose on a mobile trolley of materials wheeled into the space. The final act of the session is for the client to agree to have the picture put up on the corridor wall by pointing to where it could be placed. By this time the session is overstepping the mark – pushing for acceptance of the picture (and therapist). This did not happen on every occasion, but it did set a precedent for some external objects to be granted life, by having them up on the corridor wall.

When the client shared his own privately made drawings, they were usually of animal characters such as a fox and rabbit standing alone. It gave me the idea of 'giving them a context' by placing them into a narrative scene where they could interact, in the hope that it would stimulate engagement and acknowledge his creativity. But there was something in the appropriation of the drawings, along with the near impossibility of reproducing their character in the same way, which meant this idea became a vehicle for expressing dissatisfaction with the therapist. 'You're shit at drawing' was the message pushed under the door.

Time for art therapy

How to engage someone who avoids all aspects of being? As if resisting being born into this world – and then of controlling every aspect of their non-being. My approach is scripted: 'It's time for Art Therapy . . . here for 20 minutes, where it's possible to'.

He's holding up three fingers to indicate – 'You've got 3 minutes'. It's a near impossible start and impossible to establish the container since we're standing in different spaces, and his art materials are not present.

The experience is intimidating and deskilling. Useless. As it must be for him. His feelings not mine – but impossible to think about in that way as I stand at the window struggling to be the art therapist – not knowing how to respond to his kicking of the door with bare feet. A look so frightening it's impossible to leave behind when work finishes. Being observed on CCTV. I am filled with murderous thoughts. The only option is to turn inwards towards the art object and continue with the picture I prepared earlier.

Fragment 3

SESSION 60

At the murder scene thirty years after the terrible event, I ask the Chief Inspecting Officer if it's okay to take a picture, and surprisingly he says 'Yes', whilst looking disinterestedly along the verge of the road. I ease out my phone and take two quick pictures – too self-conscious to hold the camera straight or still. It must be the artist in me trying to get a handle on the scene; a gate into the field, the grass under the bridge has grown back and there's no sign of the struggle, the shallow river running by. More like a beauty spot than a place of horrors. I've had enough. I didn't really want to come here but they wanted to jog my memory, and I was able to provide one new piece of detail. The place where the car was parked was not how they said it was. All it did was bring back a feeling of sickness and guilt and fear, then back to work after another sleepless night.

On the approach, the client exhibits a gesture of despair – it was like this at the beginning – his non-acceptance – futility – force-fed art therapy – provoking violent self-harm – indicates with hand – not now – not today – go away – communicates to the staff by head banging on the observation window his disapproval. I reassure the staff it'll be ok. They are aware of his need for maintaining control over all aspects of his life. Mirrored by the sinking feeling in the pit of my stomach, I continue the long walk along the length of the corridor to the interconnecting door – The Art Therapy Space, holding photocopies of his drawings and a large-scale reproduction of the fox and the rabbit on the easel. I had thought myself 'clever' to develop Winnicott's mirroring technique – to acknowledge his creativity. I did not consider the appropriation (theft) of his images might never be good enough.

Fragment 4

SESSION 75

There's an axe embedded in the back door of our childhood home, some time a long time ago, but lived again when violence raises its profile to be witnessed and felt. The sounds before and after the axe struck are ever present. I am a weak useless child and it's impossible to think or speak.

The picture attracts closer inspection. He's engaging. But it's impossible to think of this as 'success'. His eyes pressed up close to the glass with disapproving looks. Circulates pointed finger to temple suggesting the therapist is not entirely present. Therapist smiles, nodding – it's not funny because this could be understood more concretely.

Presenting the colour palette, therapist asks,

"What colour could the fox be?"

Shrugs shoulders.

Therapist holds palette to door window.

He points with gloved hand at two colours with circulating finger to suggest mixing.

It's difficult to assess the direction of the pointed finger and I name the colour "mix red with yellow".

Nods approval.

When I get this wrong the result is vicious – head banging, door slamming and door kicking, sometimes forcing termination of the session.

Fragment 5

SESSION 100

There's nothing worse than following a poor leader because they will inevitably let you down by ordering you to do the most stupidly dangerous things. Delirious with thirst we set off across the desert in broad daylight when we're supposed to be hiding from the enemy. Craving for water can send you crazy and we're driving across the desert in armoured Land Rovers on mined tracks, carrying burmoils to collect water, which was sparse. The dread of having to accompany our leader. Until he finally broke down, and that was somehow a relief. Waiting for supervision. I've been here for months now, providing daily sessions. Unlike the military, I've never been sure who, if anyone, is in charge, or if anyone reads my daily electronic session notes. Some could hardly be termed 'session' since they barely survived a few moments as the violent head banging and screams of desperation brought a fearful retreat. I wonder how much of my own anxiety I'm carrying into the session and recognise my own symptoms, where the lived catastrophe is carried ahead into every uncertainty.

He's holding a handwritten message to the glass 'You're shit at drawing' – same as before. I've had enough. I write to my supervisor saying I want to end the work, but he's not available. We have a telephone discussion in the evening and the message is – I have to continue.

Fragment 6

SESSIONS 101–103

Sitting with Jonah Jones (RIP) in a hand-dug hole fortified with stones and sandbags on a mountainside in the Middle East sharing a tin of apple pudding. "Very tasty", he says, and then the incoming shells started exploding all around us – a rocket approaches like an express train and passes immediately overhead. I thought I was about to die – but it crashes to the ground without exploding. We can see the mangled wreckage – lumps of cheap green Russian tin smouldering nearby.

When in doubt or difficulty concentrate on the art object. The new aim of the sessions is to engage the narcissistic part of the client's self and provide a portrait with which to engage artistically. He agrees a series of photographic poses for the iPad – the poses are strikingly aggressive.

In the next session I manage to work on the portrait, while sometimes talking about composition and space. The client engages fleetingly between bouts of disinterestedness. He brings a drawing to the window, a copy of the photograph we took in the previous session. It's difficult to examine because I might reveal the impoverished nature of the drawing through my gaze. We plan to make a large-scale portrait on canvas.

It didn't last long. Who knows what went on in his mind? Engagement and curiosity are replaced by avoidance, fear, and loathing. He kicks the door as I approach, the message is clear – stop – go away The possibility of us working together in the group room that we had discussed now feels impossible. Applying charcoal to the figure, there's a bang at the window – I turn – he hides. Then he's gone.

Fragment 7

SESSION 120

How, when you least expect it, and when there is little hope other than death, something happens to turn it around from catastrophe to survival and that moment where all that you experienced was bad is transformed miraculously into peace, harmony, and survival. In that moment one forgets how terrible and hopeless it was. The returning helicopter has brought the Brigadier hot-foot from Empire to tell us to gather up our kit and move off this godforsaken position. Last night when the rocket landed I was thinking of dying – regretting not attending the will-making session provided by HQ, but I thought it was tempting providence and went home early. Now it's all forgotten. We're still hiding, but at least we're not overlooked by the enemy. And then the unbelievable happens. I'm in the group room setting things up when suddenly he appears walking determinedly to the entrance. He's in the room where I'm standing. I've laid a trap. A table and chair with art materials. He's accompanied by three members of staff. They stop at the door, and he enters alone. I take a seat by the table, and he starts sketching a vase of flowers.

"What you drawing?" he says.

I hold up an earlier sketch of him.

"Weird", he says.

He starts attending art therapy in the group room. It was helpful to acknowledge his creativity by presenting a written resume of the drawings and words he had used to express himself outside the sessions. Some basic neuroscience about how drawing helps to exercise and establish neurological pathways. This had the most effect since he was also wanting to get better. He couldn't understand what had pushed him so violently over the edge. The team could hardly keep up with his progress, they even started thinking of a move out of segregation.

It would be nice to think that we settled down to a semblance of a routine with him attending art therapy in the group room – but expectations never match reality. His pattern was to make progress then regress. A series of events started to take us backwards, all conspiring to regress the client. As a consequence the violence turned outwards towards staff, and soon he returned into segregation to protect himself and staff. Returning to provide art therapy through the observation window felt like a regression, and he said he didn't want to attend any more.

Discussion

The particular setting in which this work took place used an art-focussed approach drawn from the art therapy studio. Two elements are significant here. First, the use of concrete interactions around art materials and art objects as a non-threatening way of relating. We might think of this as object presenting (Winnicott, 1971) on the therapist's part. Second, the primitive feelings of extreme threat to existence (annihilation), infused with old memories of extreme states of fear and violence. The work seemed to be partly about bearing these unbearable feelings, surviving them, with the client. The consistency of the art process helped keep me going amidst immense self-doubt and allowed occasional moments of connection.

It is not unusual in art therapy that the therapist encounters interpersonal difficulties from a fearful or aggressive patient. It's quite normal in acute, forensic, and penal settings. In fact, one of the features of Art Therapy is that it provides a safe potential space for these difficulties to be worked through using art materials (alongside the therapist). We are, therefore, open and prepared for such difficulties. But to work separated from the client, in a corridor space where the patient had the choice to view (or not) from beyond the airlock that segregated us, made it impossible to create a single container – as if we were on opposites sides of a divide – which we were. In a unit where the only constant was the client himself, around whom staff and practitioners circulated, day and night, in their shifts and tasks and where it was stated many times that he 'ran the show'; where the client refused to comply and used all forms of emotional and physical attack as a way of controlling his environment, thus maintaining a sense of relational certainty (for himself). There were many attempts to shift the therapist out of role and into that of a non-operating lacuna; to be controlled and positioned, to serve other functions (than art therapy). The transference and counter transference were at times intolerable. To summon the courage to face the client and experience their murderous feelings of being 'killed off' required an internal reminder on my part of the difficulties he might have been experiencing – to negotiate and fend off such primitive feelings.

Verbal interactions with the patient were almost impossible, but repeating a range of descriptive scripts, such as 'Time for art therapy' – 'Art helps us to exercise the brain and start to feel better', provided the boundaries, function, and illusion of the existence of a therapeutic contract. The client turning up to view from the corridor window was considered 'engagement'. He did not stay long – a few minutes at the most, but enough to register his curiosity and make a gesture or comment. For the client to divert his attention from defence or attack to take notice of the picture making and point to the palette was both transformative and engaging. The simple act of curiosity was enough to confirm engagement.

Normally in art therapy the art object forms a hinge in the triangular relationship between client and therapist, but in this particular client it was as if only the picture was allowed to exist. This was object relations in its most primitive form. This is how art managed to survive. Interpersonal relating could only be experienced through object presenting.

Withdrawal from the session brought its difficulties too – experienced as a form of abandonment following the trust given by the client to engage with the picture making. For the client, a terrifying dilemma of how to relate to the therapist who will shortly pack up and leave – returning the next day to repeat the ordeal. On exit with trolley and easel through the swing doors at the bottom of the corridor – a quick look back down the corridor to see the patient standing at the airlock window observing the exit – a distant forlorn figure, contrasted sharply against an eerie pleasure of having completed the session to escape for another day.

References

Bonneau, J. (2017). The Structured Studio Setting. In: K. Killick (ed.) *Art Therapy for Psychosis: Theory and Practice*. London and New York: Routledge, pp. 90–114.
Winnicott, D.W. (1971). *Playing and Reality*. London and New York: Routledge.

12 Making art alongside each other in a therapeutic art studio

Exploring the space between us

Helen Omand and Patsy McMahon

We sit in a large, dusty workroom. It is abandoned, tranquil, and lit by the after-noon sun. Patsy thinks the tranquilness is left over from its previous occupants, who were weavers – the hours of meditative, methodical work imbuing the space with calm. The bare floorboards, where we place our artworks, are strewn with fragments of coloured threads. The room is soon to be knocked through by devel-opers who are slowly refurbishing the building, but for now we choose it as our meeting place to hold a series of conversations. Its temporary nature lends it a liminal 'in between' feeling; it is a neutral space for both of us to talk and look together at our art.

Introduction

Our conversations were the basis for this chapter, which is co-written by Patsy, a member of a therapeutic art studio, Studio Upstairs, and Helen, an art therapist who works there. Holding in mind our different roles and perspectives, we set out to explore the experience of making art alongside each other in the studio, where it is part of the ethos that staff also make their own artwork in the group. Each day at the studio is facilitated by art therapists, who are called 'studio managers', and attended by a group of regular members who come and go as they like over the course of the day. We chose to write together because, over some years of knowing each other in the studio, we had shared many conversations about our art processes and exhibited our artwork together in group exhibitions on numerous occasions.

The 'therapist' making artwork alongside the 'client' has been controversial in UK art therapy history and we wondered what effects this practice had in our studio group and on our relationship with each other. We wanted to investigate this topic because, first, existing art therapy literature doesn't often include the service user's voice directly or in detail on this subject and has been written only from the therapist's perspective. Second, we found the existing literature didn't always apply to our somewhat unconventional community setting, and we had a hunch that the role of therapists' art making would vary across settings and have a particular function in ours, Studio Upstairs.

DOI: 10.4324/9781003095606-15

The roots of Studio Upstairs are found in the revolutionary ideas of psychiatrist R.D. Laing (1960), which argued that the seemingly illogical conversations of people labelled schizophrenics were full of meaning and could be seen as a response to the madness of society, which was itself disturbed. Out of Laing's ideas The Philadelphia Association was developed with its emphasis on therapeutic communities and the importance of patients being taken seriously as human beings. Psychiatric divisions of patient/clinician, well/unwell, mad/sane were challenged and equality in interactions was sought. These influences resulted in a particular approach at Studio Upstairs, including making art and exhibiting as a community. The studio is open all day for people experiencing a range of mental health difficulties to come and go as they like. Art therapists are called studio managers to reflect that the person is not in treatment but a member of the studio community and an artist. In this chapter we use all these terms intermittently. One of the functions of the studio is to encourage people to find meaning in life through art and develop their artist identity, which is used here in its widest sense to encompass any aspects of art making processes; from our first experiences mark making and exploring materials to visiting galleries, talking about art, and organising exhibitions, which members take an active role in.

For this chapter, we chose four of our artworks to look at retrospectively together and recorded our discussions. We used an empty workroom we discovered within the ramshackle arts building Studio Upstairs is housed in, which allowed us a separate space to speak in more length and depth than in the studio group. In the discussions, more space was given for Patsy's responses than vice versa. This mirrors the delicate shifting balance of relationships in the studio: we simultaneously hold different roles, yet in making art and exhibiting alongside each other we are artists together. In writing together, we took on co-author identities, which was not always easy. Patsy said, "*I find it disturbing when emotional things are described in a clinical language. I've been disturbed by some psychiatrists putting my words into clinical language*". Several times Patsy pointed out when Helen's therapeutic language put up barriers. We had to negotiate the language we used together. We use 'third person' to distinguish between our different viewpoints and 'we' for our shared author voice.

Drawing on our conversations we first distilled some points about the function of therapists making art and some potential problems. From these, we suggest that in our setting the practice enables different identities to be held simultaneously by studio managers and members, with artist identity being a point of overlap. It is a rich meeting place where we can manoeuvre and shift roles; members sharing skills or advising and the 'therapist' bringing imperfect human aspects of themselves in their art to be seen by members. This shared identity helps flatten hierarchies between staff and members.

Second, we ask, what about the art itself side by side? Both our artworks occupy the metaphorical space between us. Skaife (2008) has suggested this is an intersubjective space, where an artwork's meaning is created between client, therapist, social context including the group and the artwork itself. What is the effect of the therapists' artworks meeting the members' artworks in the intersubjective space? We found that our artworks 'spoke' to each other, both in the studio group and anew in the shared space of our conversation. Seen together, our art brought up for us personal, social, and political points of connection; in our case, feminist thinking, being mothers, and being women artists. As well as shared experiences differences emerged too, for example, generational differences. Some were nuanced, for example, we discussed the way we identified ourselves – Patsy's working-class roots and her Irish British family's prioritising of politics and education; Helen's white middle-class English and Scottish background. There were also our experiences of art school and Patsy's experience in the mental health system. Our artworks 'belonged' to us individually as artists yet seen together brought these aspects into the space between us.

Issues provoked by the literature on making art alongside clients

Studio managers at Studio Upstairs have been making art and exhibiting with members for over thirty years now, but this has not always been a fashion-able or comfortable position. American literature has extolled the benefits of art therapists making art alongside their clients, but the practice has been relatively unpopular in the UK. Historically, Case and Dalley actively dis-couraged art making alongside clients in their first handbook of art therapy (1993), suggesting the art therapist cannot simultaneously make art and hold the client in mind. That this view persisted might explain why Helen has often encountered surprise, interest, and questions about boundaries from other art therapists. This is starting to change (see Mahony, 2011; Marshall-Tierney, 2014; Nash, 2020).

Of particular relevance to the philosophy of Studio Upstairs is the potential role of therapist's art making to help flatten the power dynamic of the therapist/ service user relationship. This is what Greenwood and Layton (1987) describe as 'side by side' working, a sense of equality between therapist and client, exemplified by the group acting as the therapist and the therapist joining in the art making. Moon (2002) also discusses the equality that it can bring; both par-ties involved in the shared creative task and equal under the gaze of the other. This has been noted too by Mahony (2011), and Marshall-Tierney who notices the power balance of 'being with' rather than 'doing to' in a clinical context (2014: 99).

However, how and why the therapist's art is used seem to depend on the set-ting. For example, in his acute setting Marshall-Tierney (2014) suggests the therapist must be prepared to have their artwork freely taken and altered by patients. This didn't apply to our community setting with its emphasis on devel-oping individual artistic identity and finding meaning in everyday life through art practice, and where there is more separateness between self and other. In some settings the therapist's artwork belongs purely in the intersubjective space (Marshall-Tierney would not take his work home for example). In contrast, Rogers's account of her own studio in a residential setting has echoes of artist in residence – artwork is hers and exhibited later; 'It is hard to say how much of my artwork was stimulated by clients' themes, how much was countertransference, and how much was my own material' (2002: 70). These ideas were useful in thinking about Studio Upstairs where we felt that artwork, somewhat contradictorily, 'belongs' to the studio manager's artist identity yet, along with members' work, can also be seen as part of the group's life. Mahony's (2011) research suggests a way of investigating this relationship visually by examining the therapist's and the group's artworks alongside to reveal the complexity of group processes over time.

We have to balance the evidence of the usefulness cited by the aforementioned literature with aspects that may be problematic, for example, clients may feel distracted by the therapist's art or experience the therapist as not fully present (Brooker et al., 2007). The discrepancy in the literature over this issue suggested to us that more communication about the role of the therapist's art making (why we are doing it, and how clients feel about it) is needed. We aim to add to this literature and help build up a picture of the spectrum of therapist's art making across settings.

Creating the atmosphere: some initial benefits and problems of making art alongside each other

We both observed that seeing everyone, members and staff alike, engaged in a creative process creates a particular ethos. Patsy found, "*it sets a kind of atmosphere of people working, without someone specifically saying do this or do that. It's saying it's okay to do artwork. It's not saying it but demonstrating it*". This puts art first and brings about an atmosphere of shared creative endeavour and absorption.

Bearing in mind the aforementioned literature, Helen wondered if there were unhelpful aspects that it might be harder to discuss. We talked about managers being trained in art and how it might feel if managers make skilled work in front of members. Patsy pointed out the nuances to this, "*It depends how you do it. If it's showing off, that's different to being inspired by seeing someone really involved and absorbed in their work and doing it well*". Helen was curious about whether envy in the studio might show itself via art. Patsy felt,

> *You wouldn't be human if you didn't occasionally envy someone, but I think it's not specific to member versus manager because there's a very wide gradient of skills amongst the members. Some people have not done art before, and others have been to art college.*

We acknowledged that it was hard to stay with feelings of frustration if something wasn't turning out how you wanted, this might be exacerbated for members who haven't done much art before. However, we felt that feeling dissatisfied and struggling with a creative process is a shared experience for members and managers. Managers can voice their difficulties or indecisions as they work to model something about the uncertainty of the process. Members and managers can often be overheard saying, "Oh, I'm not sure about that bit", or we might have a moment where we really don't like our work and consider throwing it away or starting again. Making a piece of art involves tolerating the unknown as we don't know where it will go. It is a risk to commit a mark to paper. It is useful to get other people's opinion on the work too. For example, what colour might work, or when is something finished? Members comment on Helen's art, sometimes critically, for example saying, "Don't overwork it!". Seeing the therapist as a complex human being involved in an uncertain process with all its benefits and frustrations is levelling. The roles we play in the studio shift about, and skill sharing is common. Members can teach managers techniques or advise. The back and forth lends an equality; we are in a shared struggle with art.

Turning to the art: 'the tit power temple'; mothers and therapists in the studio

Patsy chose her Talking Breast sculpture (Figure 12.1) as the first artwork we would look at. The interactive sculpture is a large breast made of expanded foam. Inside is a little motor linked to software on a laptop, which drives a snake-like light around to a rhythm. Patsy described it:

> *It was supposed to be an asp like Cleopatra's breast. It had a speaker inside and a recording of me saying 'I'm glad you came come to consult me as you did when you were young'. It was about early memories, memory before speech, before we can talk. Someone helped me with the technical bit, I wanted people to walk in the room and then the breast start talking. I exhibited it at Stoke Newington Library. At the exhibition I did a workshop with it too, with the help of my two daughters (Figure 12.2). The breast invited participants to make a breast from clay or record their earliest memories and each of my daughters, in their twenties, led one or other workshop. I called this The Tit Power Temple. I promised I would make a later artwork playing back the recorded memories with people's clay sculptures of breasts. I later exhibited this at an exhibition in a derelict house in Peckham. The first workshop was very successful and generated a lot of excitement.*

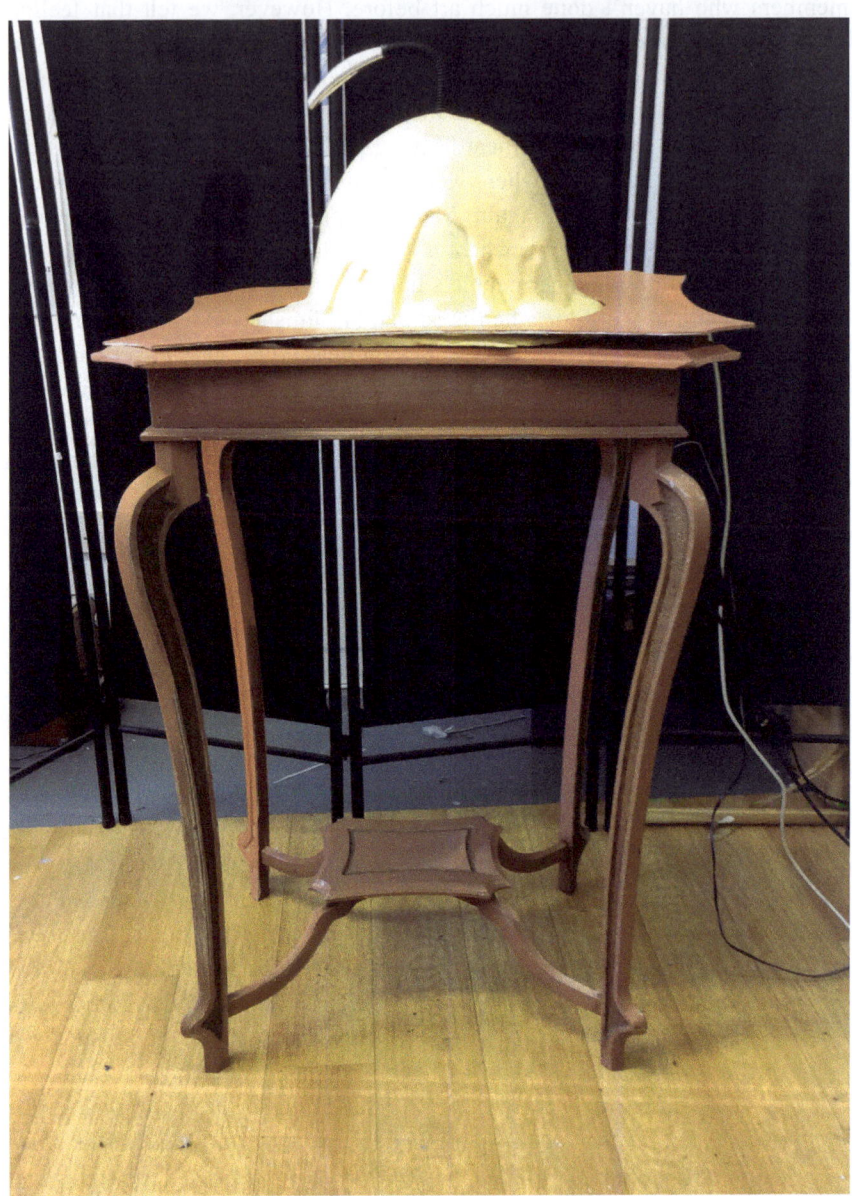

Figure 12.1 'Talking Breast', by Patsy McMahon in exhibition at Stoke Newington
Library.

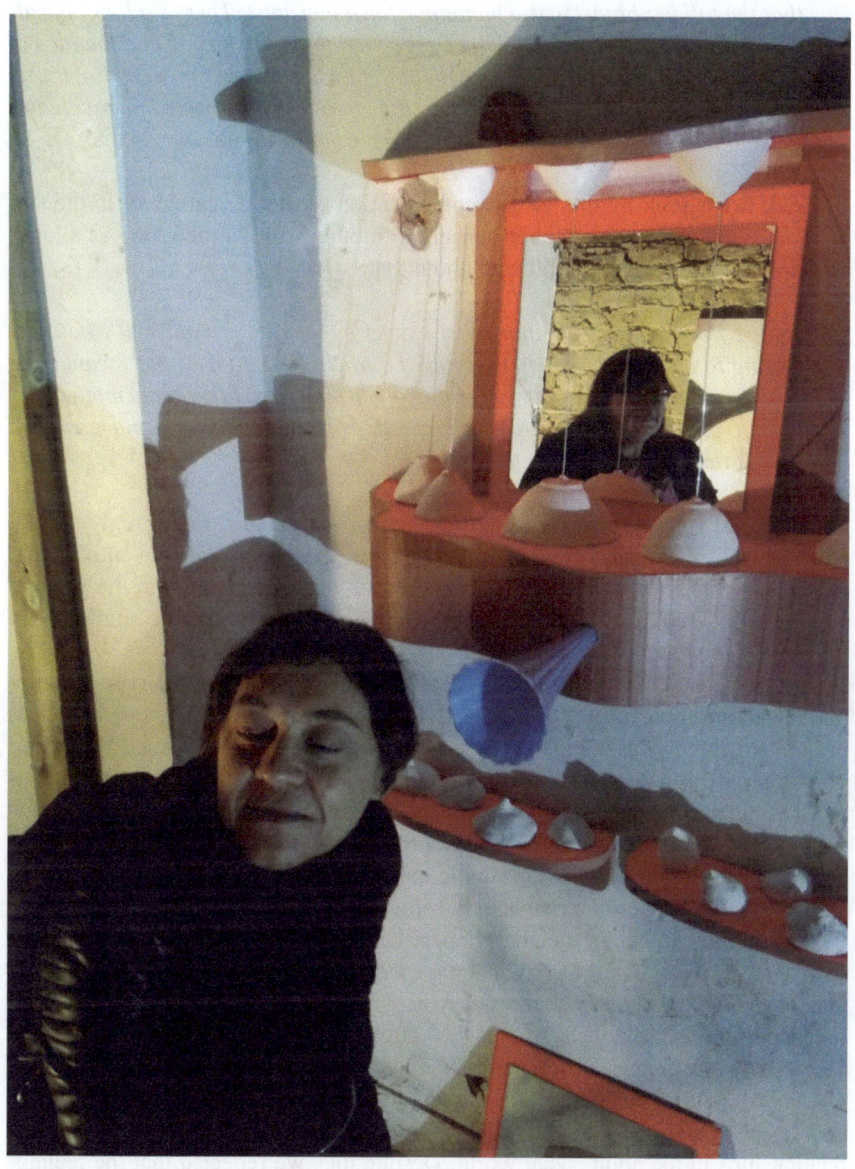

Figure 12.2 Interactive workshop installation by Patsy McMahon.

Helen asked about the presence of the breast sculpture in the studio. Patsy said,

> *It took a good while to make, and people were interested. It occurred to me that the talking breast was a metaphor for a therapist. There's a lot of parallels with therapists and mothers in psychoanalytic thinking. I had the idea of this breast as providing a place you can go where there's no moral outrage, you are who you are, no judgement. But there's also a period of psychiatry and childrearing that blamed the mother for an awful lot.*

Helen was struck by this visual representation of mother/caregiver in the studio and asked whether Patsy herself held a 'mother' role in the group as a long-standing member. Patsy wasn't sure about that,

> *I don't think it's a good thing that even I'm seen as a mother, it's not very freeing to always be seen in that role. I quite like it in a way, but I want to be free for people to see me as something other than that. I think as a mother you have to carve out some space for yourself, from all the demand and need, and I think that's important for the child too.*

The breast sculpture suggests nurturing, protective aspects of caregiving, but Patsy's artwork had also brought up for us gendered expectations of 'mothering' in a patriarchal society: these themes came into our conversation in the present, and we wondered how ideas about 'mothering' also came into the studio group via Patsy's artwork.

The conversation prompted us to recall the image of Louise Bourgeois' sculptures with multiple protruding breasts. These images of disembodied breasts brought to mind irresistibly for Helen the psychoanalytic concept of the 'part object' breast as a way of relating, to mother or therapist. Mulling over Patsy's words, that mothers needed to 'carve out some space' for themselves, Helen wondered if her own artwork was sometimes a way to find space away from the demands of being a therapist/symbolic caregiver and look after her own needs, amongst intense seven-hour days in the studio.

How might that feel for members? She asked Patsy, "*Have you ever felt excluded or neglected when a manager's attention was on their artwork?*" Patsy had felt that, once or twice, when managers were heavily concentrating on their artwork for longer periods, but said if she wanted their attention, they would leave their artwork. "*Sometimes a manager has said, can you hang on a minute? And you can. We are all grownups*". Within our therapeutic community framework, it seemed important that people could negotiate with the manager and each other to get their needs met, like relationships in the adult social world. Despite this, we reflected that the feelings it might bring up, of being neglected or out of mind, might echo powerful feelings from early childhood, which could be acknowledged or explored. The extracts from our conversation show how Patsy's artwork brought up these themes between us: it made visible, in a playful way, ideas about preverbal early feelings and their connection to adulthood and asks, what do we expect from 'mothers'?

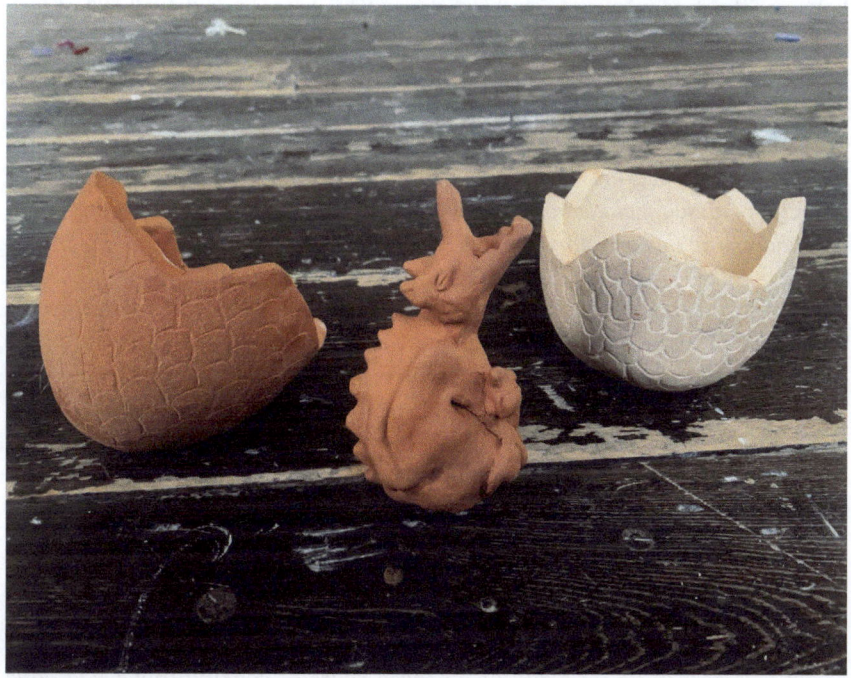

Figure 12.3 'Dragon's egg' by Helen Omand.

An ongoing process: constructing meaning in the intersubjective space

The following example suggests how an artwork accumulates layers of meaning in each new space it inhabits, which can be useful in different ways. Helen brought her artwork of a clay egg, containing a dragon, for us to look at (Figure 12.3). When she made the egg there had just been a major shift in Studio Upstairs' structure. Two groups of members had been amalgamated into one group, and Helen was working with a new co-therapist, and everyone was struggling to come together. Helen said,

> *Whatever is happening in the studio at the time seeps into my artwork. I made the eggshell pieces separately from different clays and they dried too quickly. I spent days sanding them down, trying to get them to fit together (much to one member's amusement who is a trained ceramicist). I realised my struggle with the materials embodied the desire to make things 'fit' and the reality of the rather painful process the group was undergoing.*

Later, a conversation started with a member who associated the two different halves of the dragon's egg with skin colours. This brought up the subject of race in the studio:

> *We spoke about two black members of the group who over the past year had lost their funding to attend, which had changed the representation of eth-nicities in the group, I became aware there were more white members of the group, myself included as a white therapist. There was a need to think about addressing this imbalance and their loss for the group.*

The artwork made unconscious material in the group visible in the studio, which helped studio managers reflect on it verbally with members.

We now opened the clay egg and considered it together. Patsy said,

> *Looking at your artwork now, I like the dragon in there. I like the surprise of it. It reminds me of something that I'd forgotten about. When I first broke up with my partner, I'd been in a mental hospital and I'd been homeless, and I finally got a flat after I'd been in a hostel for nine months. I didn't want to do any cooking in the kitchen, so I made artwork in the kitchen instead. I made a cast, with wax, of this frog and I filled it with blue vinyl. When I cracked open the mould this blue frog popped out. And it was sort of like a birth, of all these years of cooking that I had done and everything, and it was just so momentous that moment. I was in the kitchen, and it was so liberating to be doing artwork, because my partner never encouraged me in that direction, never made any space for me. It's interesting that reminds me of that. The crack, and suddenness. It was a similar size.*

We were struck by Patsy's visceral associations to the work and how the sensory qualities of size, weight, shape, evoked vivid unexpected memories. Patsy noticed the egg is broken which suggested a 'patching-up' and felt there was a parallel with how when women break down, psychiatry 'patches up' women, often sending them back into the same broken domestic situation. Previous themes of women's emancipation that had arisen with Patsy's breast sculpture were evoked, and we felt this was an example of how our artworks 'spoke' to each other in the intersubjective space of our conversation, accumulating new meanings as we talked. They brought up shared points of reference; the power of making artwork for oneself, taking up space as artists at home and in the studio and preconceived ideas about gender and domesticity. Patsy observed, *"I think women in general have been brought up to be more considerate and think about other people more. There's both positives and negatives to that especially as an artist"*.

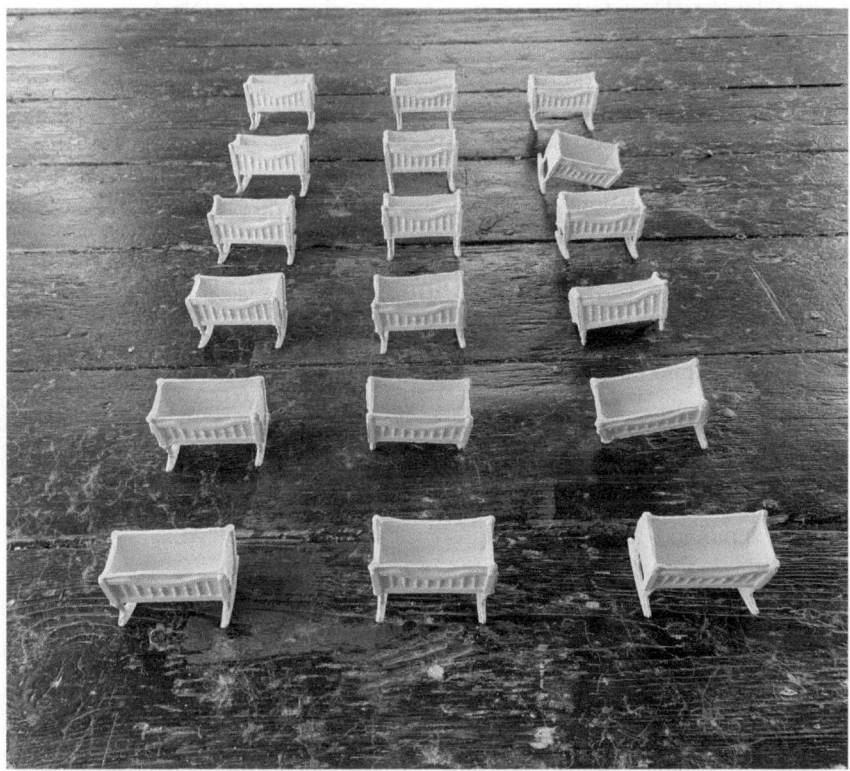

Figure 12.4 'Cradles' by Helen Omand.

Contradictions: where does the work belong?

Helen asked if there was a particular piece of her artwork that Patsy remembered her making. Patsy said,

> *There was a piece of your artwork which affected me a lot. I'm thinking about the one with the little cots. It took me back to when I was very little and I was in a nursery. They left us in these cots for hours on end and I remember being bored to tears. It was just after the Second World War and there was not much good childcare available. My mother was not aware of how neglectful they were and we were very short of money. She had to work as we were very reliant on her income. Luckily at home the atmosphere and care of us was good. I found it quite helpful looking at that work, because, I don't know why, it just brought up the feeling of this, but without it being . . . you'd done the work very carefully. Looking at the rows of cots helped me think about a painful experience but without trauma.*

Helen felt that there was no fixed meaning to her artwork, it was available to be related to by members, to start conversations and explore experiences. This was unpredictable as there was no way of knowing what might be evoked in another, as Patsy's response shows. It might be tempting for an art therapist to stick to neutral themes, but in this context we felt studio managers needed to bring more of their artist selves and develop work that was meaningful to them. Art can be fanciful, surreal, or horrifying; it can show our 'disturbed' aspects in a sublimated, transformed way, different to acting in a disturbed way or acting out.

The cradles artwork (Figure 12.4) did not actually originate at Studio Upstairs, somewhat controversially (she felt), Helen had made the mould in another setting and then brought it into Studio Upstairs to cast more cots, use the kiln and develop them into an artwork for exhibition. Helen had wondered in supervision where the work belonged – where was the boundary with her art practice outside of Studio Upstairs? Once present in the studio, the multitude of cots suggested a group and evoked other responses, for example, the nursery. The artwork developed a new life in the studio and the casting process generated interest in mould making, but perhaps it remains a grey area. This may differentiate Studio Upstairs from other settings as the art therapist's artwork is further along the scale towards personal art practice (Rogers, 2002) and further away from being a type of response art (Nash, 2020), although how far will probably vary between individual therapists and their approaches. We suggest the artwork belongs to the therapist's artistic identity but draws its meaning from each intersubjective space it inhabits – in the group, in exhibition, and here later in our joint conversation.

Last reflections: from the studio and into the space between us

We next chose a series of eight paintings by Patsy 'Archetypal poses' (Figure 12.5 shows three). We spent time arranging these on the studio floor. We debated hanging them, but Patsy decided she liked looking down into them, like pools of colour. She described them,

> *I had some pictures of ancient Greek plaques and one was of a procession of people in particular poses. I got my daughters to dress up and position themselves in the same way and I photographed them in my mum's garden. When they stood in these poses they evoked particular feelings. It was a special, kind of magical day, in my mum's garden.*

Helen vividly remembered Patsy painting them and conversations arising in the studio group about play and people's childhoods. In the making of these paintings, involving three generations of women in her family, Patsy interwove her identity as an artist with her identity as a mother, drawing on one to inform the other.

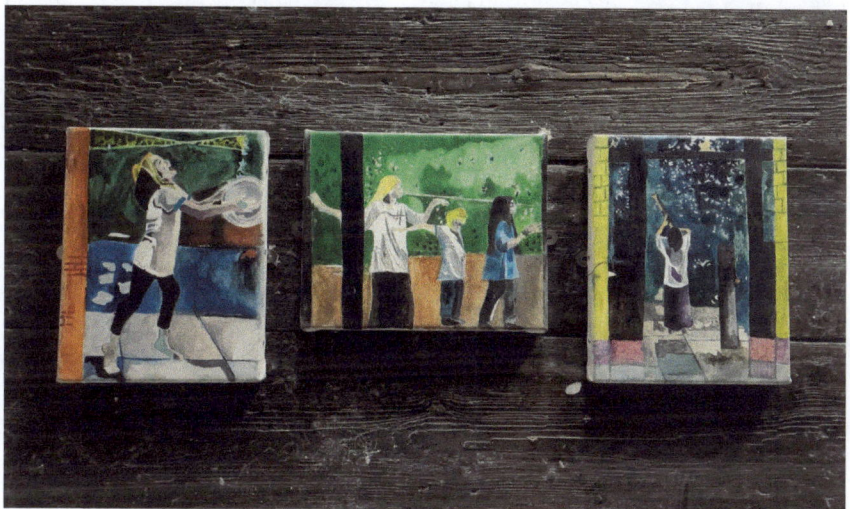

Figure 12.5 'Archetypal Poses' by Patsy McMahon.

Discussing them we spoke about motherhood. Helen had been pregnant while working at the studio and so members knew she had children; there is a visibility to pregnancy as a public life event. We observed that although we did not speak together in the studio group about our experience of being mothers, our artworks related or 'spoke' to each other. We noticed for this chapter we had chosen artworks, in response to each other, that referenced motherhood and childhood. This may also unconsciously reflect the generation gap in the intersubjective space between us, with its echo of mothers and daughters.

Conclusion

Patsy commented that at art school tutors never revealed their own art practice, "*it was sort of shrouded in mystery*", leaving a sense that there was an aspect of themselves they weren't revealing. This preserved the teacher's role and the power dynamic. At Studio Upstairs, managers making art helps shift the power dynamic and artist identity is a shared point of overlap. In this meeting place shifts in roles happen. Patsy said, "*You can negotiate hierarchies in the studio because they are more undefined in a way*". Therapists, in trying to make work that is meaningful, are seen engaged in uncertain processes, struggling with art. Complex aspects of themselves are shown, a far cry from the all-knowing 'expert' clinician.

In the context of the studio group, we found that the therapist's artwork can make visible the preoccupations of the group. However, in our community setting it also 'belongs' to the therapist as part of their artist identity. The art object can hold these simultaneous and contradictory positions as it accrues many meanings.

We explored our artworks in the context of our memories of the studio group – but recalled retrospectively in our dyadic conversation in the empty abandoned workroom. We unconsciously chose our artworks in response to each other; other members and studio managers would clearly have brought in different aspects of themselves and their artworks to the shared space of the conversation. Our artworks brought into the space between us personal, social, and political points of connection and difference, and we wove new strands of meaning between them as we looked and talked.

References

Brooker, J., Cullum, M., Gilroy, A., McCombe, B., Mahony, J., Ringrose, K., Russell, D., Smart, L., von Zweigbergk, B. and Waldman, J. (2007) *The use of artwork in art psychotherapy with people who are prone to psychotic states: An evidence-based clinical practice guideline*. London: Oxleas NHS Foundation Trust and Goldsmiths, University of London.

Case, C. and Dalley, D. (1993) *The handbook of art therapy*. London: Routledge.

Greenwood, H. and Layton, G. (1987) An out patient art therapy group. *Inscape: The Journal of the British Association of Art Therapists*. Summer, pp. 12–19.

Laing, R. D. (1960) *The divided self: An existential study in sanity and madness*. Harmondsworth: Penguin.

Mahony, J. (2011) Artefacts related to an art psychotherapy group: The art therapist's practice and research. In: Gilroy, A. (Ed.), *Art therapy research in practice*. Oxford: Peter Lang, pp. 231–251.

Marshall-Tierney, A. (2014) Making art with and without patients in acute settings. *International Journal of Art Therapy*, 19 (3), pp. 96–106.

Moon, C. H. (2002) *Studio art therapy: Cultivating the artist identity in the art therapist*. London: Jessica Kingsley.

Nash, G. (2020) Response art in art therapy practice and research with a focus on reflect piece imagery. *International Journal of Art Therapy*, 25 (1), pp. 39–48.

Rogers, M. (2002) Absent figures: A personal reflection on the value of art therapists' own image-making. *Inscape: The Journal of the British Association of Art Therapists*, 7 (2), pp. 59–71.

Skaife, S. (2008) Off-shore: A deconstruction of David Maclagan's and David Mann's 'Inscape' papers. *International Journal of Art Therapy*, 13 (2), pp. 44–52.

13 Terms of engagement

Aspects of facilitating open art therapy groups for adults in a psychiatric inpatient setting

Annamaria Cavaliero

This chapter considers the way art therapy is delivered in an acute inpatient setting via open groups on wards. It describes different routes to, and ways of engaging in, these groups by patients who are experiencing psychosis. The chapter reflects on aspects of participation and the particular role agency plays in an environment where people often feel at their most helpless. It explores the complexities of running open art therapy groups for people who are acutely unwell and distressed in a challenging environment and provides vignettes from clinical practice. All names are changed for reasons of confidentiality.

It is fitting to set the work within its context of a National Health Service (NHS) setting in a London borough whose demographic has one of the highest incidences of psychosis in the country and which is heavily impacted by the austerity of recent years and historic issues to do with poverty and social deprivation, such as housing, employment, and education, as well as issues with immigration and legal status.

There are probably only a handful of bespoke art studios in psychiatric hospitals still in existence and these may not even be available to art therapists but reserved for artists from the community. The spaces where art therapy takes place now are often in multipurpose activity rooms. It is important to think about the studio model in art therapy and how it developed in the medical setting before changing into the different form it exists in today. In 1946, two years before the inauguration of the NHS, Edward Adamson joined Netherne Hospital as an artist and set up a studio for patients (Adamson, 1984). Netherne was still running on asylum lines at that time. Adamson provided patients with their own workstations and offered art materials, but otherwise he did not teach or interpret the art made. This work had a large impact on the development of art therapy in mental health settings. Jumping forward, Killick talks about a studio in a converted ward of a psychiatric hospital, which was described as 'church like' or a 'sanctuary' by those who visited or used it (Killick, 2000: 102). It had been an art studio since the 1960s, and it was used by inpatients experiencing acute psychosis to make art in, or simply to sit in and was generally considered a safe space. Killick has written and edited many papers on the subject of art therapy and psychosis and the importance of the physical setting (Killick, 1997, 2000, 2017). Wood (2000), in discussing the significance of studios, stresses the importance of having a place in

DOI: 10.4324/9781003095606-16

which a person experiencing the flooding of unconscious material that psychosis unleashes can find a sense of absorption and creative reverie. The studio 'exists on the border between the therapist and the institution' (2000: 43). Brown (2008) reflects on the studio both as a physical space, which offers the possibility for different processes to take place and as a 'transitional object' between the concrete and the symbolic and between inner and outer realities. Referencing Bion, Killick reflects on how 'the art room played a crucial part in mediating the experience of a containing object for patients in unintegrated states of mind' (Killick, 2000: 101). Bonneau writes about the structured studio, an approach developed by Killick, as the site in which 'the artwork as body 'part' is placed in relation to the 'whole' of the art therapy setting by means of its boundaries and the negotiation of possibilities and limits in relation to the context' (Bonneau, 2017: 98). All agree that the setting is a very important component of relational art therapy.

It is important to note that the studio settings described earlier are dedicated rooms – similar to the artist's studio – where evidence of the artist(s) remain in place when the sessions are over. The art therapy groups I describe need to be set up and dismantled each time of use, leaving no trace of the activity that has been going on for the length of the protected group time of one hour. The art therapist sets up tables and chairs and puts out a large variety of art materials and paper for participants to select from. All participants are invited to reflect with the therapist and/or group about their imagery. This can happen at different points in the group. Due to the varied presentation of participants, I make decisions during the group as to whether group looking and reflection time are something that could be tolerated that day.

The Art Therapy service where I work mainly offers open group sessions on acute psychiatric wards. The rationale behind offering sessions on wards is to be inclusive as not all patients are able to leave the ward environment. The sessions are open because of the awareness of the active features of psychosis that can impede involvement in a more formal closed art therapy group. Patients may feel aggrieved at being detained under section and thus very mistrustful of anyone or anything associated with the hospital, they may find it difficult or alarming being with others, they may be very restless and agitated, or conversely very sleepy and tired. The effects of medication can directly impact their affective states. By offering open groups the therapist can invite patients to engage in the group on their terms. The therapist's job is to make sure that the sessions start and finish on time, thus holding the space for the patients to make as much use of as they are able.

All patients are welcome to make use of the open group unless it is deemed unsafe. The therapist personally invites all patients each week just before the session. There is no formal assessment process, and the sense of a therapeutic alliance is not clear. Nevertheless, the therapist must try to establish this alliance with the groups and the individuals within it. This is often best achieved by modelling something for the patients. This might mean holding the group open for the patients whether or not they choose to make use of it, tolerating repeated rejection of an invitation, acknowledging, and accepting a patient's need to leave the space. Sometimes it can mean sitting in an empty room with difficult and powerful feelings of shame, uselessness, and rejection while also trying to be open to the chance that patients might join the session at any moment. At times it can be a volatile space, full of comings and goings and energies, when it is difficult for the therapist to think. A concrete example of modelling is the therapist's capacity to tolerate disturbance – material may emerge in the art making or the behaviour and communications of the patient that is hard to bear – the tolerance is demonstrated by the therapist consistently turning up for sessions and keeping to the time boundaries. Qualities that are crucial to this role are persistence, resilience, and flexibility.

In a classic open studio setting, there are usually work benches and easels and areas that a person can make into their own workspace as well as shared tables. In the rooms where I work on the wards there is often only enough room to have two trestle tables pushed together to create a large table. In some rooms there may be a separate table or work bench. Interestingly, I have noticed that the majority of participants choose to sit around the table even when alternative workplaces are offered. Apart from introducing patients to the materials the sessions are non-directive. The therapist sits with the patients as part of the group but is able to think about what happens from a psychodynamic perspective.

Challenges that face the ward-based art therapist are often to do with the institution itself; there are rapid changes in the ward composition from week to week, this means that there is little or no chance to prepare before the session. Patients may be presenting with different degrees of severe psychopathologies – mainly psychosis or the extremes of mood disorders. As the participants all come from the same ward environment this will affect the process; antipathies and affections may have been formed outside the group. I think of the role of the therapist in the open group as being a consistent, non-judgemental, and empathetic presence whose job is to facilitate a creative space as well as to witness, attune, and think about what is being communicated, both on a conscious and unconscious level.

There can be all sorts of ways that people approach the open groups. For some it is straightforward, but for others it may be daunting. I have noticed that for many it is a tentative process, a dipping in and out of the space. I think of this kind of engagement as a dance, involving an approach, almost a dalliance, then a retreat before an actual commitment. Sometimes a person will enter the room ostensibly for another reason, perhaps to look out of the window. This may be a way of testing what it feels like in the room and might help them to join the group next time. I've experienced a patient coming in and placing things in the room, a cup on a windowsill here, a book on a shelf there. This went on for a period of weeks until he finally came in and joined the group and made very good use of it. I thought of these cups and books as transitional objects (Winnicott, 1971). By leaving them in the physical space he may have felt he was leaving something of himself there, thus assisting him in his journey to physically joining the group.

All doors on psychiatric wards have a clear glass window for safety reasons. Often patients will walk up and down the corridor outside the room, glancing in as they pass. My sign on the door welcomes all patients and often they will come in. On other occasions, patients may delay their attendance in the group with concrete reasons and come in for the last fifteen minutes. This may be a way of managing how much time they are ready or willing to spend in the group. Sometimes I notice people actually rocking on the threshold of the group, leaning their bodies in while their feet remain outside. To cross the threshold is a huge step. As a therapist I feel it is important to acknowledge this, to create a welcoming-enough space, and to encourage people in but not to expect them to cross the threshold until they are ready. When you stand on a threshold you are hovering at a point of choice. It is not necessarily a comfortable place to be. But making a decision to carry the body across a threshold is an important act of will and agency.

Bick's paper 'The Experience of Skin in Early Object Relations' (1968) discusses a stage prior to Melanie Klein's model of splitting. She notes how the skin functions as a boundary in object relations, serving to bind the different parts of the personality together. For this to happen, the infant must first introject an external object capable of doing this for them. Bick suggests that only once this has happened is the infant able to fantasise internal and external spaces. We can think about the art room as a container whose walls (skin) separate the inner world of the creative space from the outer world of the ward. It can be containing for patients to be creative in the safety of the art therapy frame; the therapist is there to hold this frame in an attentive way, s/he will let them know how much time there is left until the session ends, pay attention to what is being made, notice demeanours, do their best to attune to how individuals are feeling and make any necessary adjustments. This is akin to what Bion (1962) describes as *maternal reverie*, a calm state of mind that promotes the mother's repeated capacity to receive and transform distress into comfort, which is key to promoting a similar capacity in a child throughout life.

The word threshold moreover implies a liminal place, existing on the border, neither in nor out. This can symbolise the position in which many psychiatric patients find themselves – psychotic illness can lead to family breakdown, the inability to sustain employment, studies, or friendships, and people can feel marginalised and become isolated. The grasp on reality is tenuous, certainly different from the majority, inside and outside are not clearly distinguished. It is hard to be in a world that has a different perspective from your own and that rejects your thoughts and feelings as delusional. The art therapist might also occupy something of a borderline position in terms of their relationship with the medical model. While the therapy room, transformed into an art studio by the art therapist, is in and of the ward, it can simultaneously feel outside and not of the ward. Entering the space means crossing into something very different from the medical environment.

Foulkes (1964) saw group therapy as a means of flattening the hierarchy of therapist and client. It is relevant that art therapists undergo extensive group and personal therapy during training and beyond, they carry this experience with them into the therapy room; this is an area where therapist and patient share the experience of feeling vulnerable and being exposed but also of being seen and heard. The open studio group invites each participant to engage on their own terms although one of the aims for the group is to encourage inclusivity through side-by-side working, in an atmosphere of creativity and reverie. But the group is also open to whatever the patients might bring and that can include disturbance, frustration, anger, and distress. Art materials can be used to externalise and release these feelings too and allow them to be thought about.

Although it is an open group it does need to be defended against interruptions from outside forces, the group needs to be an oasis within the ward that is not affected by the practicalities of ward life. How the art therapist offers the contradictions of both an open group and a group that is closed to interruption is an ongoing and delicate task.

At his recent exhibition *In Real Life* at Tate Modern (2019–2020), Olafur Eliasson placed a sticker with the word 'threshold' near a door to an outside space. Next to this he placed another sticker saying, 'there is no outside'. In both his studio practice and art exhibitions, Eliasson poses the notion that inside and outside are dynamically related (Dincer et al., 2019). It is hoped that in the non-directive art therapy group participants can access their inner worlds through using the art materials. The group, with its frame of time boundary, room, art materials and therapist can allow participants time and space to focus inwards. The title of Eliasson's exhibition is also pertinent, as people experiencing psychosis have no doubt been grappling with the stress of 'real life'. Bonneau thinks about psychoses as 'an escape from the irresolvable dilemma of 'being-in-the-world' and the limits that entails' (2017: 91). A threshold also has to be crossed to leave the group, the ward, the hospital (all important rings in the circle of containment for patients), and rejoin 'real life'.

An example from my experience is Thomas, a patient who had recently been discharged from the ward. He soon returned to hospital as a voluntary patient after realising he was not feeling well enough to be at home. The return to the real world had been too soon, he was not ready to be in the environment he normally felt safe in because his internal state was still one of agitation and disturbance. In art therapy he was only able to articulate this by making an image (Figure 13.1). He told me the safest place he knew was at home in the living room with his family. It felt very sad that this place was not accessible to him at this moment. Did he literally feel shut out? After we explored this verbally, he returned to embellish the image. The addition of the recycling bin seemed significant. Might his rubbishy feelings be recycled into something else – a different way of being-in-the world? In the ward, bizarre behaviour is less noticeable than it is in 'real life', and this removes some of the stress of managing day-to-day life. Over weeks he continued to come to the group, quite often making two types of images in the same session – an abstract image as well as an image of himself accompanied by text. He used these drawings to illustrate how he was feeling. Both ways of working seemed absorbing and important for him.

As patients are admitted to the ward and each patient adjusts and settles into its rhythms, so the group finds its momentum like a boat on the waves. As patients start to reconnect with their sense of self, so their engagement with the outside world begins. This may affect how they use the ward group, whose membership ebbs and flows with the movement of admissions and discharge.

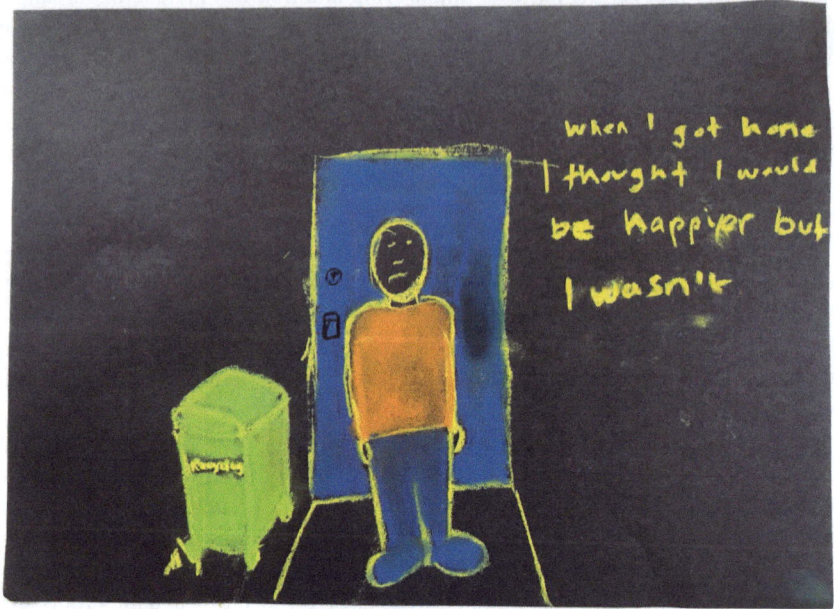

Figure 13.1

How does the therapist manage this discontinuity? S/he stays aboard the boat and cannot see beyond the horizon. This can be sad for the therapist when the patient has been an active member of the group. There is not always a chance to say goodbye or have any sense of an ending. Working on an acute ward means managing one's sense of expectation and celebrating the small connections. The boundaries of the group extend to the care of the artwork made in sessions. Folders that are stored by the art therapist can be experienced as a way of living in the therapist's mind beyond the time limits of the session or indeed the admission.

Foulkes (1948) stressed that the group therapist must be equally attentive to what is happening in the individuals and in the group, and I would assert that this is the case in open groups as well as closed groups. The ward-based art therapist needs to not only be attentive to both the art making process and the dynamics of the group but also to what might be going on outside the group, for example, if a patient is called out of the group to attend a meeting or ward round or if the patient has recently been in one of these. They may have just received news that a tribunal has not gone the way they had hoped, they may have been asked to take medication against their will, they may have witnessed a fellow patient being restrained, or have received bad news. All this information, some of it gathered from an earlier handover, has to float freely in the therapist's mind.

If we think about psychosis as a defence against unbearable feelings, then it may be very difficult for a person in its grip to be receptive in groups to the distress of others, especially if their emotions resemble those that are being actively defended against. Lucas (2009) talks about a patient who fell asleep in groups, seemingly under the influence of his antipsychotic medication, however, it was noted that after the groups he would play badminton energetically. His sleepiness was then understood as the patient mimicking the side effects of medication whenever emotional topics were raised. In open groups participants can leave the group at any time. It can be useful to note what might have been happening when a seemingly engaged participant suddenly decides to leave the room. It can help shed some light on what is disturbing for this person. It is also important to hold in mind that internal processes such as hearing voices can so profoundly disturb patients that they feel the need to leave a session.

I find it helpful to bear in mind Winnicott's (1971) ideas about the child and its relationship with caregivers, where he reflects on how the mother's face is the first indicator of another's mind. Participants often look to the therapist, perhaps for some reassurance or attention. In a quiet absorbed group, when participants can focus and engage easily, I consider the effect of the art therapist's presence as that which might foster this quiet and absorbed practice – Killick describes using a 'persistently interested yet objective approach', creating a 'safe place for the patient to *be*' (Killick, 2000: 104–105).

However, we have to accept that the therapist's attention may not always be welcome or settling at all, and it may be that this is affected by the power dynamics of race and class, where a therapist might occupy a potentially powerful and persecutory position in the mind of a patient. The following example helped me to appreciate this: during a group a young black woman, Raquel, looked up and addressed me but when I responded she said, "Don't look at me with those glasses!" Later she again asked me something but when I replied she immediately pushed me away with words. My glasses seemed to represent something persecutory to do with the power of the therapist, not just looking but looking with 'those glasses'. Perhaps they served to duplicate my act of looking. It made me think about how the therapist can, perhaps unwittingly, occupy a disturbing position. It is important to think about how the white therapist may be perceived by the black patient and to accept that this can bring up many feelings around oppression. The delicate work is finding a way to reflect on this in a meaningful way with patients.

Interpersonal dynamics can be worked with in various ways in art therapy groups. In an open group one of the participants, Sarah, really wanted to voice her feelings about not knowing why she was in hospital nor who was responsible for her admission. On more than one occasion she said that she would rather be dead than languishing in hospital. Another participant, Josefa, was using the art materials chaotically and Sarah turned on her in an irritated and abrupt manner. Josefa responded by looking at her hands which were covered in yellow chalk. She then spread this chalk on her paper saying, "I'm fading". Then she used dripping water to represent tears. I drew Sarah's attention to this, and she was moved to apologise to Josefa for snapping at her. I thought about Sarah saying she would rather be dead and Josefa imagining herself fading. Josefa was expressing hurt feelings but was also imagining a sense of dissolving into nothingness, thus enacting the sentiments her peer was expressing. The open group model allows both for group interaction and for introspective working. The therapist is able to move in on occasions to voice observations if necessary. If participants can tolerate some reflection on the imagery made in the session, this invites an opportunity to make a conscious connection to what has been expressed.

I often think about whether people are able to 'settle' in the groups. For some people, there needs to be some testing of the environment and the therapist. They need to know whether the therapist and the group can tolerate their distress. In order to discover this the environment may be subjected to the extremes that the patient is feeling. This might involve some confrontational behaviour. By reflecting on this without judgement, it is possible that something deeply intolerable is contained for the patient and a sense of connection made. An example of this was when a newly admitted patient, Lydia, joined a ward-based group which was already underway. She ignored me and started drawing; the atmosphere was seemingly calm with everyone in the room engaged in art making. Nonetheless, I felt on edge; after a while this patient looked up and accused me of doing nothing, of being smug, of waiting to make a clever interpretation, of creating a 'particular time' to make art which was 'incredibly patronising'. I felt my heart rate increase as a sign of fear but decided I needed to acknowledge how disturbing the group seemed to be for the patient by asking her if she wanted to talk about this. She told me how she had been brought into hospital against her will and that she had been working as a teacher before this happened. I reflected on how patients often think of me as a teacher rather than a therapist despite the lack of teaching that goes on. This may have been very painful for her seeing as she had just been removed from her professional role. After this, the atmosphere lightened and at the end of the session she acknowledged that she had felt a need to test me to see if I was really capable of seeing her as something other than a patient. I realised that what had on the surface appeared to be a calm and focussed art making session was in fact an extremely agitating experience for this patient due to the power imbalance and perceived role reversal.

The group process can also be a gentle route towards reality testing. In another group a patient, Céline, who had also been in denial about being unwell, wanted to make a self-portrait; I noticed she was looking at a photograph on her phone and thinking about copying it. After a while she put the phone away and instead started to draw an abstract piece using a variety of media. When she had finished, she spoke about this image as representing herself, there was a flat orange line at the bottom of the page, a jerky blue wandering line in the middle, a pink circle in the top right-hand corner, and red corners framing the whole image. She explained that the flat line at the bottom was herself when she was well – literally her base line – and the jerky wandering line represented her current agitation and difficulty sleeping, she said the pink circle represented her family, and we noted that the red corners might also relate to other containing factors – possibly the therapy space itself. She had in fact produced a different kind of self-portrait. The act of making the image helped her realise something about herself that she could then put into words.

People can use the art materials however they wish in the group as long as it is not unsafe to themselves and others. Not everyone uses them in a traditional way. For some it can be a sensory experience; all the paints are non-toxic. A patient who presented as mute started by making prints of her hands and feet and gradually started to use the digits to make paintings rather than just prints. Her choice of colour and mark making was extremely communicative and she was able to convey many feeling states this way. People might use materials to express overwhelming feelings, I have noticed people using water to wet and flood materials and it can be helpful if this is commented on and acknowledged by the therapist. Some people write outpourings of words. I try to think about what each product might be expressing and have accepted into my care sodden parcels of folded drawings, torn shreds of paper, sheets of paper holding only the most fugitive of marks and small thumb-pressed petals of clay or plasticine. These are often the most poignant of pieces, laden with feeling and meaning which cannot be articulated any other way, embodied objects that require the utmost care.

I hope this chapter sheds some light on how even those experiencing the severe and debilitating effects of acute psychosis can access and make use of art psychotherapy via the open group model. I have observed how taking part in the group can have a positive impact on patients' mental functioning, emotional well-being, communication, and creativity. How people engage within the space helps the therapist attune to each participant. The setting seems to allow for a kind of reflection and engagement with self and others that can be surprising and enlightening. There are challenges to the art therapist in sustaining a sense of worth in the current climate of rapid admission and discharge, particularly in an era when quantitative data analysis does not necessarily pick up the nuances of psychodynamic art therapy. How to measure the work remains challenging. I think that the key to this work, to return to the beginning of this chapter, is that engagement occurs on the patients' own terms at their own pace, within the frame of the open group. They are always welcome, always invited, but the terms on which they engage are their own.

References

Adamson, E. (1984). *Art as Healing*. London: Coventure.

Bick, E. (1968). The Experience of Skin in Early Object Relations. *International Journal of Psychoanalysis*, 49, pp. 484–486.

Bion, W. R. (1962). *Learning From Experience*. London: Heinemann.

Bonneau, J. (2017). The Structured Studio Setting. In: K. Killick (ed.) *Art Therapy for Psychosis: Theory and Practice*. London and New York: Routledge. pp. 90–114.

Brown, C. (2008). Very Toxic – Handle with Care. Some Aspects of the Maternal Function in Art Therapy. *International Journal of Art Therapy*, 13(1), pp. 13–24.

Dincer, D. I., Brejzek, T. and Wallen, L. (2019). Designing the Threshold: A Close Reading of Olafur Eliasson's Approach to 'Inside' and 'Outside'. *Interiority*, 2(1), pp. 43–61.

Foulkes, S. H. (1948). *Introduction to Group Analytic Psychotherapy*. London: William Heinemann Medical Books Ltd.

Foulkes, S. H. (1964). *Therapeutic Group Analysis*. London and New York: Routledge. Accessed through Kindle edition (2018).

Killick, K. (1997). Unintegration and Containment in Acute Psychosis. In: K. Killick and J. Schaverien (eds.) *Art Psychotherapy and Psychosis*. London and New York: Routledge. pp. 39–51.

Killick, K. (2000). The Art Room as Container in Analytical Art Psychotherapy with Patients in Psychotic States. In: A. Gilroy and G. McNeilly (eds.) *The Changing Shape of Art Therapy, New Developments in Theory and Practice*. London and Philadelphia: Jessica Kingsley Publishers. pp. 99–114.

Killick, K. (2017). *Art Therapy for Psychosis: Theory and Practice*. London and New York Routledge.

Lucas, R. (2009). *The Psychotic Wavelength*. London and New York: Routledge.

Winnicott, D. W. (1971). *Playing and Reality*. London and New York: Routledge.

Wood, C. (2000). The Significance of Studios, *Inscape: The Journal of the British Association of Art Therapists,* 5(2), pp. 40–53.

14 Family residential art therapy studio model

In discussion with a parent and member of the open-studio group

Kristen Catchpole

It was ALLLLLL so alien, but I guess for the first time, in the world, I wasn't the only weirdo. I can't remember what you said back then but something made me think that art therapists were a bunch of weirdo's too – but they liked that they were weird.

(Bobbie: a parent recorded in discussion, July 2020)

Introduction

Bobbie is a mother with learning needs who undertook residential family assessment and was a member of the art studio in the centre where I worked. She agreed to have a conversation with me to discuss and reflect back upon her parenting assessment and her process in the studio. Bobbie left the centre nine years ago to care for her child, Natty, full time. We have remained in contact over the subsequent years. Natty is Bobbie's first and only child.

The rewards of Bobbie's use of the studio highlight the need to invest in families at the point of crisis. I argue that full and considered assessments best create care packages of support for families who have learning needs. The studio can provide a vital space for families to grow and learn together, for the emergence of autonomy, agency, and the development of a capacity for decision-making in the individual. Providing specialised support for such families at an early stage is better for communities and the best use of government funding. Also, I assert that therapeutic input has, in this setting, seen a halt to people repeatedly producing children to replace those who had been born and removed previously, in a cyclical process of loss.

Bobbie and I each had a differing perspective of the studio group from our very different positions. I am the privileged one, not only because of the power bias in my favour as I was employed in 'an assessor role', but also while I have a diagnosis of dyslexia that I deem an advantage in seeing the world, she holds a diagnosis of autism and mild learning disability, and she has been judged (in the formal sense of the word) 'less able' as a result of it. We both are from similar working-class and socio-economic backgrounds. I have the intellectual capacity to have created and used opportunities to move into a financially stable position in

DOI: 10.4324/9781003095606-17

the working population. Bobbie's focus remains on childcare and living within the benefits system of financial support. Bobbie identifies as white British. I identify as a woman of Eastern heritage, although I am also seen as white. Bobbie was aged twenty-one at the beginning of her assessment and I am ten years senior.

The art therapy studio at 'Tarrington House', the centre where the work took place, had a unique role in the practice of assessment for families. The organisation assessed families; mainly parents who were at risk of permanent separation from their children. We worked with family solicitors, the local authority, and child advocates in a court-ordered process. Families at risk were placed for assessment because they were struggling to safely parent their children. The populations that I will describe have a diagnosis of a learning disability and often hold a secondary mental health difficulty. It was identified that learning-disabled parents lacked the opportunity to fully access such a complex assessment process from their local authority, hence the need for the support that Tarrington House, as a non-statutory organisation funded through legal aid, could offer. The art studio space is one aspect of the assessment process.

In my ten years of employment there I was witness to huge and challenging changes in policy with funding reductions that led to diminished access to resources for families to receive support during their court proceedings. In a short space of time, the potential for a family to access specialised assessment was reduced in time from twelve months to between six and twelve weeks.

I am acutely aware that 2005, when my employment began at Tarrington House, was a time before the banking crisis of 2008 and the austerity measures that followed in the UK. Tony Blair's Labour government was in power, and the economy was stable. As I write, in 2020, during the COVID-19 lockdown, it is currently understood that we will be living in an economic downturn, the largest seen since the Second World War. Much of my career has been spent working during economic recession and I am tainted by my experiences of the dismantling of services. While I am keen not to present a rose-tinted view of times of 'better' funded projects, I have greatly benefitted from working with other art therapists who had, within working memory, held studio models in the old 'asylum' way. I hope that the value of learning disability and mental health services will return to priority funding, and indeed they will need to, in response to the current social and economic crisis.

All names and locations have been changed to preserve anonymity.

The model

Family assessments were based on the functional and intellectual abilities of parenting. Specialised risk assessments, parent skills development, and therapeutic provision were the core processes of the practical and psychological evaluation. Multidisciplinary teams collaborated to build more nurturing relationships between child and parent. Up to twelve months was afforded for those undertaking court-ordered assessment to build skills and safe parenting practices. This length of time afforded greater understanding of the complex ways in which each family had historically functioned (McGraw, Shaw, and Beckley 2007). The aim was to ascertain a family's ability to grow and learn together and explore whether parents had capacity to safely and effectively provide a loving home wherein the children can thrive. This information was reported back to local authority social work teams and the court, with recommendations made for the judge to consider.

This population of learning-disabled parents, with mental health needs, had experienced alienation and marginalisation. Wood writes in 'The significance of studios' of how studios support what has been lost of oneself at times of distress,

> Absorption is the opposite of alienation. When alienated it is as though we stand beside and watch ourselves with uncomfortable self-consciousness. In contrast to this, when we are absorbed, we are engaged in the moment, absorbed in our lives and in what we are doing.
>
> (Wood 2000: 40)

The therapy in the studio provided a space where people would come together to share issues of oppression, difference, and marginalisation (Blackwell 2000; Malis 2017). The arriving parents presented with distress, confusion, and disorientation. All were deeply afraid of having their children removed from them again.

As such, I was hell bent on creating a studio space where the process could be user led, so their concerns would have space to be processed through art making; it was a place for discussion of the political and the proceedings that were taking place. I suggest that such a studio model offers containment and can be a location for the emergence of a person's difficulties leading to self-discoveries.

The studio was also used by its members as a space for integrating their learning from their assessment. The art objects made would provide containment of that learning for the parent's growing self-awareness and a means for collective reflection. Participants could be seen to develop self-management and the regulation of intense feelings, which was important for both the group process and their developing capacity to parent.

Like other studio models, there was not a preconceived agenda within the space other than to promote thinking and reflection. Participants were invited to find and use art materials, making sure to respect the works of others and engage with the views of others in the space, as they saw fit, while attempting to articulate their contrasting views without 'acting upon' them. All members would be considered in the group and therefore when speaking, members were invited to talk so that all might hear. The studio's facilitators, including myself, did not make art.

Bobbie offers,

> [W]hen you are actually with the art materials and you can just, like, 'look' at yourself. . . . well of course I just knew it was a good way for me to really. . . . as you would say 'process' (said laughing playfully). The studio was so important to me. It was different to the rest of the house, where I was being watched all the time.
>
> (Recorded in discussion July 2020)

The setting

Tarrington House was located in an old Manor, whose structure spans different centuries. From the driveway's lengthy approach, one is met by the large sixteenth-century timbered exterior; the shape of this elevation and its interior rooms are determined by the timbers that were obtained from shipwrecked boats. Rather than providing heat, its multiple large fireplaces acted as dens for the children, which were covered with sheets held up by broom handles or chairs, in interesting arrangements (perhaps unconsciously driven, the children often acted out scenes of pirating narratives). The kitchen areas, though fitted out with modern fixtures, were later editions in the seventeenth and eighteenth centuries. The various floors of this sprawling building with its higgledy-piggledy rooms housed psychologists, occupational therapists (OT's), speech and language therapists (SALTS), as well as support and administrative staff.

The art therapy studio was located in a Victorian conservatory flanked by greenery around the many large windows. Overlooking the central courtyard to the house, it was a secluded and quiet place. It smelled deliciously of paints, wax oil pastels, cartridge paper, baby lotion, and lush warm earth. This was a dedicated space and not used for other meetings. I worked three days a week and when I was not there the studio space was held by a SALT and a long-standing member of the support team. The time boundaries for the studio to be open were 12 noon to 10pm, otherwise it was locked (shutting for dinner between 5pm and 7pm).

A parent's decision to attend was based on a discussion with their support team and myself. Largely parents self-referred, expressing their desire to be creative. At any one time we would be working with 9–14 families. Often, the studio would be used in the evenings because the care of the children during the day took precedence. Parents' time in the studio would include the use of child monitors (audio or visual monitors of their sleeping children); the sounds of the babies or toddlers were continuous in the space. At times of a baby needing soothing and attending to, they too might join the studio group while their parent worked with the art materials.

Bobbie: case material

Bobbie had Natty removed from her care at birth. This was based on her diagnosis and local authority concern around the suitability of their return to Bobbie's mother's house from the maternity ward. The house was deemed to be unsanitary for a baby to live in. Bobbie reports that whilst still under the effects of anaesthetic she was asked to sign documents that determined her child was handed over to the local authority. Bobbie remembers that she had not known what this meant at the time. It was deemed in the high court that Natty had been removed without due diligence. After undertaking a court process of fourteen months during which time Natty was in foster care, Bobbie moved into the Tarrington House assessment centre and Natty a few days later.

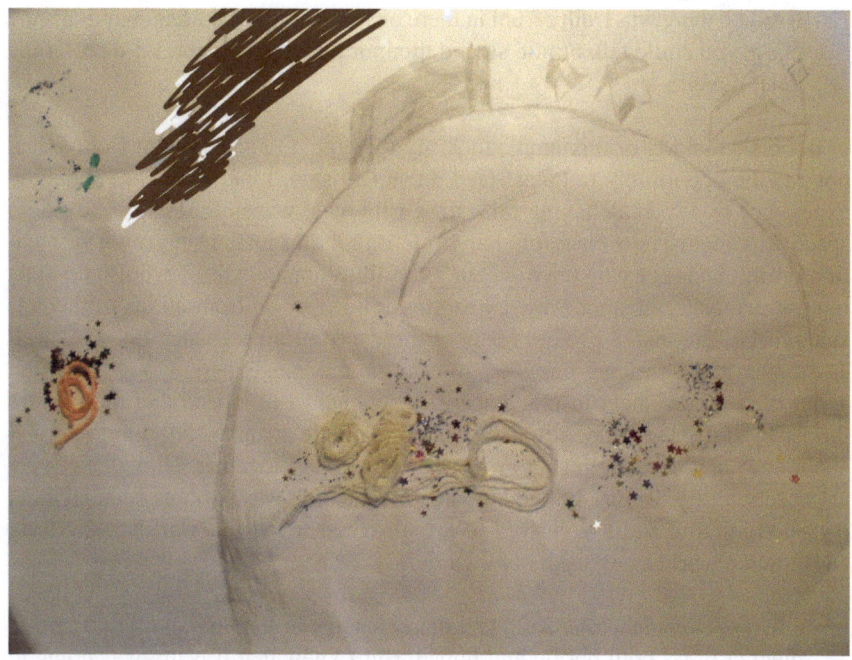

Figure 14.1

Natty did not present with a learning need, nor with social or mental health difficulties and did not require a referral to the Tarrington clinical team. Today, she is a thriving fourteen-year-old.

Bobbie selected artworks to include in this chapter, which demonstrate her development and internalisation of her process towards being the parent and person she understands herself to be today. The following are some selected edits from a recorded conversation that took place between March and July 2020.

B: The struggle is, you are pleased because you have a chance with your baby but at the same time you are really thinking, can I do this? I now have my baby, I argued for that in court. No question did I love her, of course, she would always be my world. But in reality, I was petrified.

K: I am reminded of this piece (Figure 14.1) that you made on your arrival. A spontaneous sharing occurred and words were put to the images for many people that evening. You were able to talk about having a huge mountain to climb on assessment and that you could see there being many physical blocks to the process. Another resident wondered with you if there would be many emotional blocks too. I suspect that many studio members could see their own feelings at work in others art creations, but I wonder how you think about this today.

B: God yeah, you would always be called out on your bullshit in the studio, it was like there was truth serum in there or something. No hiding, but that's the thing, you could talk or not, sit and think or not, make or not. I did prefer the quiet though.

Bobbie's making of this image took my thoughts to consider that Bobbie had not had the opportunity to breast-feed. In supervision, I had wondered about the experience of a woman having milk for a baby who was not present. The studio space was regularly a place of shared mourning and loss. In my own rumination on the image, I wondered whether the little orange ball of wool with stars represented Natty in some way. I was mindful of growth from uterus to the outside world. The image evoked ideas of the curve of a pregnancy belly, as well as the breast. When the group were musing on the image there was a discussion about their predicament in this place of assessment and indeed that their future family lives depended upon it. This helped facilitate a conversation in the group about how they were feeling and what they had to face together. These ideas were engaged with by the group members in a melancholy way. Bobbie seemed quite detached initially and I wondered to myself whether she felt worlds away from Natty, and a world away from her own family.

B: Oh, don't get me wrong Kris, I regularly hated you at points and found assessment at times both boring and horrid. But I knew that if Natty was going to go home with me I had to take every opportunity to do what I could. But actually, this was not so much on my mind when I could make art and quite frankly there were others I needed to think about like the other parents in the studio. But I guess that's it, we weren't separate, but we were, we were a group of people making art alongside each other . . . to be honest, we were all in the same boat, the authorities had taken our children and it was like, well, it was almost easier to be real because we all knew the same fear, the same horror. What could I do? I couldn't kick off with anyone because what would they (other parents) say, 'you couldn't even keep your own girl?' None of us pulled that card. So, when you have a mutual respect that everybody needs support, everybody felt pain, everybody was scared – then you sort of have your level. And you need to work; work on being a parent, grow up and be together and learn together. I had to be me so I could understand better how to learn to be a parent. No-one else would know what it was like other than those parents together in that room (studio). No one took the piss. There were disagreements, sure, but no-one was impossible.

Many of Bobbie's later pieces involved thinking about her identity as well as finding 'a meeting point' with her daughter, often her artworks would include her daughter's name and a word of introduction; there seemed to have been a shift.

B: I had to admit to myself that I needed help with certain things. When I arrived at Tarrington House I had just lost my dad. I was in the process of thinking

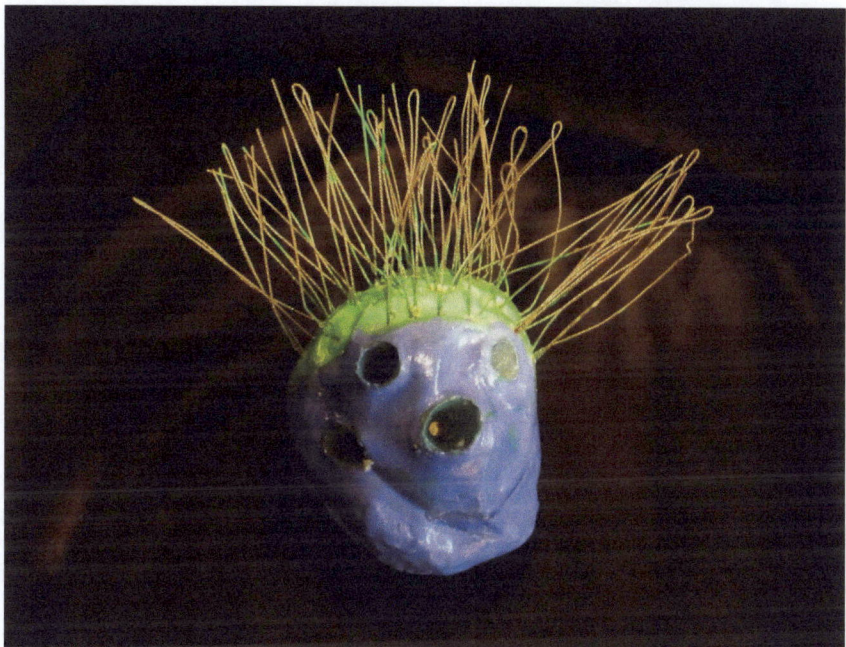

Figure 14.2

about being a daughter to my lost dad and our strong bond and that loss, and also trying to work out who I was as a mother. That's what the piece was about when I put the wires into my head in the sculpture (Figure 14.2). It's quite hard to look at again now, but at the time I needed to know what my head was doing, like, inside.

Through this piece, I could see that I was allowed to be angry at death, especially when I was embarking on a new life with Natty – a new life my dad would not be part of. I was angry Natty was taken. I was angry at my Autism, which was me and in me but apart from me at the same time. You know I'm not even prototypical autistic, I just find people and organising tasks really hard. I was angry that it was also a time for me to come out. As a gay woman I could see that there was difficulty ahead too.

In one studio session, because Natty couldn't sleep, she came down to join Bobbie and they spontaneously made a piece together (Figure 14.3). Bobbie was stabbing a piece of clay prior to Natty's arrival, and she sat Natty on her knee to look over the art materials that she might like to use. Natty saw the plastic tool as a mother bird feeding baby birds in a nest. Natty then proceeded, under Bobbie's gaze, to draw a nest and two birds in flight. Earlier in the day, they had been exploring nature together in the garden. My immediate association to the birds in

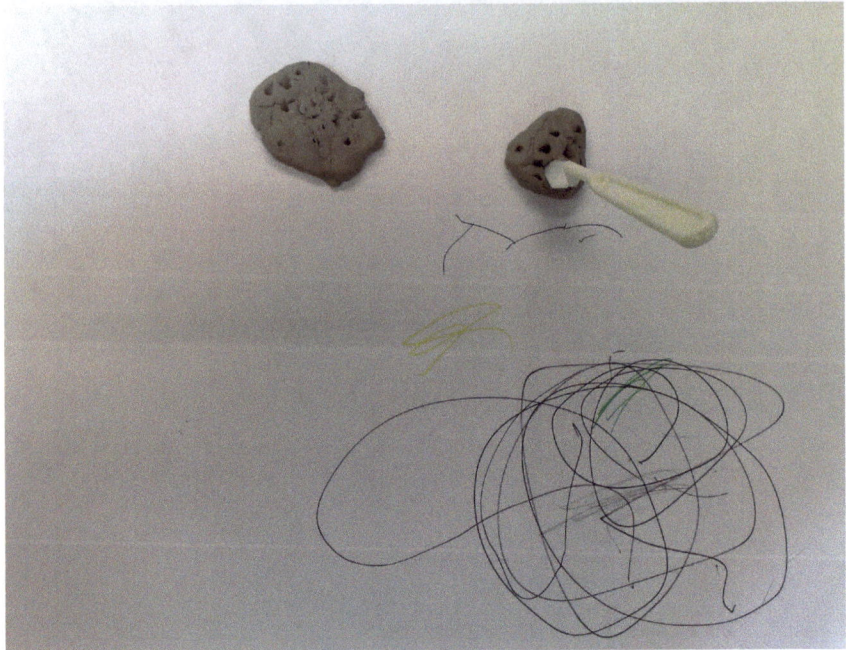

Figure 14.3

flight was Bobbie and Natty getting ready to fly the nest of Tarrington House; then as sadness crept upon me via the transference, I wondered too about Natty's loss of her foster parents. In this representation, was Natty attempting to understand where her carers had 'flown to'? Working with the metaphor, it would seem that Natty was well able to bring an important narrative into the work with her mother and after the months of Bobbie working to find a way to be with her daughter, Natty also found a way to be with her mother. At this point through the residential assessment, Bobbie could take joy in Natty, giving kisses and cuddles of warmth to her as they giggled and laughed on their shared chair. At the time, the group were inclusive of Natty's arrival to the space and as a community recognised the children as 'ever present' members of the studio.

Discussion

When I have worked with parents engaged in their own art making process as part of a group, I have witnessed significant changes to their functioning, parenting personhood, and capacity to think. I found that my ability to enter a state of reverie (Bion 1961) in the studio correlated to the member's capacity to find and build reverie with their child, whereby there could be appreciation of individuation, so that a parent could build an understanding of their child in their own right.

Both parent and child could use nurturing relationships to develop into their own being. It was not unusual to see enmeshment in the initial parenting dynamic presentation; often, the delicacy of the work would involve creating time to consider 'needs' and to appreciate the challenge of the demands of their children.

In this case, even though Natty had been removed from her mother Bobbie for the first year of her life, it became possible for them not only to be reunited but also to then live as a family and to thrive for the next twelve years; this is ongoing.

Much as the studio provides and allows for the mess of creativity, and metaphorically the messy nature of processing one's own feelings, so there seemed to be further capacity to build-in tolerance of a child's 'messiness' (O'Brien 2004). Initially, Bobbie struggled with Natty's messy eating and would discuss the onerous task of tidying up after her. Over time, I felt there was a direct correlation between Bobbie's growing ability to be with her own mess in the studio (alongside others processes of making and being) and to develop the capacity to position herself in an experience that meant the task of tidying up was a creative one, because Natty was learning and through her messy food-tray was also an artist in the making.

Natty 'finding' a sense of herself through her 'food work' and the reverie of the shared experience of being together in this discovery meant that the 'tidy up time' was seen as a time for internalising what had gone before. Bobbie was learning who Natty was, and learning that newness, discovery, creativity, and nurture, along with the anxiety that comes from being in relationship, the 'mess', was an invaluable way of Natty and herself being together. These transferable happenings and transformations were not limited to this example. When mum had an enriched inner world of her own and thinking time in the studio, she became increasingly available to her child. The studio space, much like the tidying, is not only practical it represents an ordering, attentive process.

The studio model provided an accessible space to parents where vulnerabilities could be worked with and, in the main, diminished. Art materials were used to explore and contain an internal process that paralleled their learning and change in a creative way (Nolan 2019). This space was possible because there was reliable funding, a fairly stable population of families in the house, with a stable multidisciplinary team around them.

Subsequently, due to policy changes, local authority funding squeezes, and the ending of Legal Aid, the time in the studio and the space itself was lost. Towards the end of many years of working at Tarrington House, assessments were restricted to six-week initial assessment interventions. This drastically reduced the provision and process that had been available to families, a process that regularly led to their learning how to live together safely and lovingly, a capacity that almost entirely mitigated the need for fostering and adoption services. I consider that assessments inclusive of the studio model are far more economically viable for local authorities, government, and society. With thoughtful support and shared parental rights, birth parents and children can then remain together, thus lessening the possibility for a drive to seek relationship through repeatedly bearing more children, to continually fill the place that the loss of the previous children has left.

My purpose here has been to represent and speak to the value inherent in supporting children and learning-disabled parents to stay together wherever that is securely possible. At Tarrington House, the therapeutic provision within the studio model was a crucial part of this process.

References

Bion, W. R. (1961) *Experiences in groups and other papers*. London and New York, Routledge.

Blackwell, D. (2000) And everyone shall have a voice. *Group Analysis*, 33: 19–20.

Malis, D. (2017) Crafting the visual voice: Art as agency in studio art therapy. *ATOL: Art Therapy Online*, 8 (1). Available at: https://journals.gold.ac.uk/index.php/atol/article/view/438/pdf.

McGraw, S., Shaw, T. and Beckley, K. (2007) Prevalence of psychopathology across a service population of parents with intellectual difficulties and their children. *Journal of Policy and Practice in Intellectual Disabilities*, 4 (1): 11–22.

Nolan, E. (2019) Opening art therapy thresholds: Mechanisms that influence change in the community art therapy studio. *Art Therapy, Journal of the American art Therapy Association*, 36 (2): 77–85.

O'Brien, F. (2004) The making of mess in art therapy: Attachment, trauma and the brain. *Inscape: The Journal of the British Association of Art Therapists*, 9 (1): 2–13.

Wood, C. (2000) The significance of studios. *Inscape: The Journal of the British Association of Art Therapists*, 5 (2): 40–53.

Part III
Curating, exhibiting, and archiving

15 Looking at the curation of art made by older adults in a median art therapy group

Kristina Page

Introduction

This chapter is based on my experience of running a slow open median art therapy group with a studio-based approach, in a community setting for older adults. The group has run for over ten years and has accommodated a slow turnover of therapists and members.

What may be unique to this group is the monthly arrangement of a 'viewing', a named process of group members' artworks being hung on the wall of the space we work in. Group members then come together to talk about the artworks *as a group process*. This is the only time the group is in dialogue together and is in notable contrast with the couplets, triads, or subgroupings that interact throughout the rest of the month. The viewing has developed in different ways in relation to the different therapists, and since I took on the group I have always aimed to hang the work myself, as I understood in the handover that this was to be part of my role.

Part of this viewing process highlights the differences in looking up at the work on the wall rather than down on the floor, when thinking about communications 'from the works' that may contribute to the group dialogue. My intervention as curator may be something of a visual 'rearrangement' of the group, which may impact where we look, and I will explore this further.

Outline of the group

The studio model of the group means that members, although expected to arrive and leave on time, are given a certain autonomy with regard to how they use the space, the materials, and myself. The tables and chairs are pre-set up in two long rows, with chairs that provide sixteen places. There is an opportunity for individual (and when requested, confidential) attention between the therapist and a member to take place, otherwise members are equally free to use the space to make work, without any verbal exploration or interpretation of process and/or product.

The potential for building relationships between members within the group can be impacted by group members also meeting one another in pairs or subgroups both during and outside of the art therapy group. These meetings may be in other

DOI: 10.4324/9781003095606-19

activities held within the project itself, therefore, the service itself can act as an outer boundary. Sometimes there will be a subgroup who go together for tea following a session; as the group does provide tea and biscuits this can be thought about as a refusal within the group, which may create a split between those who can take from the group and those who use the group to possibly re-create a feeling of frustration or inadequate care; of needs not being met, which may echo other relational structures. (This idea of refusal may also be felt within the viewing; either as a resistance to speaking about the work, or by speaking but avoiding any curiosity from other members which may aim at making a personal connection.)

Because the group does not hold a circle of chairs, but rather is set as two long rows, the physical movement around the room can become a psycho-geography, where people stop at different places in order to meet different needs during the two hours. Interest in each other's work leaves a trail, creating patterns of movement; there are places that are more frequently visited than others. The provision of a sink, kettle, and tea making invites interactive 'waterholes' that can be stopped at for many reasons. These 'communicative processes' Stacey (2001: 221) can be imagined visually as a looping or like a comma, part of the complex group interactions. By stepping back, a member has the opportunity to redirect their focus by socially interacting, looking at work done by others, or find a way to potentially escape difficult feelings or emptiness brought on by not knowing what to do. By feeding oneself, taking in tea/coffee/biscuits or conversing, feelings can be avoided or buried.

The idea of looping or pausing that is part of the group session may also be experienced in the way the work is looked at during a viewing, where patterns of physical movement can be explored, mixing interior and external worlds through the dynamic mix of the images. Once on display up on the wall, certain works may invite one to come in, create connections that could unintentionally form a 'visual subgroup' through colour, subject matter or size, or equally may suggest one keeps their distance. If an image is central it may be 'visited more often' with the act of looking, some images may become 'resting places' for the groups' eyes; similar to the tea making hub, where one returns due to the familiarity of style mixed with a pleasing image. Where one looks may depend on how each viewer seats themselves, in close proximity to their work or far away, or perhaps preferring to sit near a friend as priority, disregarding the physical space in relation to their own artwork. For those with short sight, it may even be impossible to see the work; leaving only size and colour to be identified.

Curating and curatorial bias

The word curate stems originally from Latin, meaning 'to take care'. Although this may not be how we associate the act of curating, in this chapter I am offering the connection with curating as an intervention that may have a positive effect when thought about and acted on. This could echo the idea of making links verbally through connecting one member to another through a growing understanding of the development of group dynamics.

A curator works with, and handles, the artworks individually from the art-ist, therefore the fact that members give me their work, which I physically hold and take away to hang, could be thought about as a physical intervention. This becomes a physical interrelationship between myself, members, and the artworks. I become part of the relationship with the work, in contrast to if works were hung individually by members, which would keep the therapist's involvement separate echoing the style of art therapy groups where members will place their own works on the floor, in whichever way they choose.

Curating in art therapy is described in depth by Reagan, who has presented a clear and concise argument for the employment of curatorial practice. She points out that by placing artworks together, the 'shared concepts' and 'unex-pected connections' can generate meaning; 'curators put artworks in conversa-tion with one another' (2017: 30). She argues for the use of curating as a tool for art therapists and includes the idea of developing trust in the non-linear process of art.

In my experience, during six years of studio-based art therapy with this group, the careful placing of one image next to another can be experienced as a thera-pist's comment both on the artwork and on the individual. It can be taken person-ally and cause a range of emotions. There will always be a work at the centre and another at the edge; even the positions of 'far right' or 'far left', high or low will become part of an unconscious processing.

The viewing begins with each member choosing an artwork that they wish to show. This can be current, or older work from their portfolio. Lasting about forty minutes, the viewing takes place sitting on chairs where the members look across and sometimes upwards towards the work. This has a physical impact on the dynamic between art and viewer, and because we sit, the art-works look down at us. In this move from making to talking, the transition can seem difficult, and it is interesting to question whether there is a sense of feeling smaller when the 'gallery' is up, a line of images that may be look-ing expectantly back at us, and a feeling of not-knowing, as if there was an expectation or desire that we did know, that each of us understood the work, and knew how to speak of it.

Inter-visual dynamics

The content that follows, of what is said, what has or hasn't been said, or who has felt listened to, heard, understood, or ignored, can all connect with the life of the artworks and their concrete presence. The organisation of the artworks on a wall may create a viewpoint for each artist as they reflect on individual pieces that may sit one under another, side by side, or at the far end, far away from the artist themselves. All these positions are open to dialogue and may provoke some sort of response regarding the placing of oneself socially within the group and internally connect to self-esteem. The artworks may critically mirror ideas of being 'centred', 'self-centred', or 'off-centre', or 'beside oneself' and 'on the edge'. Even the gaze of a member itself may require turning the head to the left or the right, if not face to face with one's work. A large bold artwork may silence and overshadow a smaller one, much like in a group dialogue there can be silence, and this may mean many things; so also a work that dominates might be hiding an inability to communicate personal material.

Changing the viewer's viewpoint by emphasis on a work that may seem to hide by its fragile marks may open up new thoughts and potential relating. This is relevant in that some of the members are dealing with the deterioration of their sight, or hearing, or both. Lack of seemingly sufficient healthcare due to long waiting lists for this client group, the social stigma of the 'elderly' can feel echoed in the lack of provision of decent quality materials. This can mean the work relies on hope and maybe some imagination; against my wishes I feel the cheap materials and thin paper could be carrying a message through me from the outer container of the project, which could then impact from me to the group. This message can be thought about as 'it doesn't matter'. If this attitude of 'it doesn't matter' is carried over to how the artwork looks, it may also suggest a level of disposability, which could then be internalised back into group members' self-esteem. Does it matter then if the paintings aren't hung well? As one may prompt a silent group member with curiosity about the silence, the dynamics of refocusing our attention can bring to the centre what may remain otherwise on the edge.

Thinking about aesthetics

The aesthetics of art in art therapy have been explored by Henley (1992), who suggests that there may be preferences of the therapist that may compromise empathic regard. In hanging the work, I aim for aesthetic balance where works lead into one another. Some works are bold, large, and may dominate. How would a dominant figure be thought about within a verbal group, and would the therapist find some way to make room for nuance and fragility, so there is a chance that more can be heard? Although within a verbal group this orchestrating could be held as a group responsibility, I suggest there may be a certain conducting occurring as one can only listen to one voice at a time, *whereas in a viewing all images are seen simultaneously*. It is like a group mirroring a group, yet the mirror has been adapted and directed perhaps to flatten potential hierarchy amongst the members and create resonance. The opportunity to point at a unique artwork can bring attention and provide an experience of feeling seen.

In *'The Object Stares Back: On the Nature of Seeing'* Elkins describes looking as hunting, but he suggests it is the object that is the hunter, and the viewer that is drawn in, their eyes being caught by a detail that acts like a 'hook'. He writes: 'All seeing is heated. It must always involve force and desire and intent . . . There is no looking that is not directed at something, aimed at some purpose' (1996: 21–22). He suggests there is no looking without a desire to possess. These words are powerful. There is something in them that resonates in me when the members sit looking and I wonder what they are looking for. By my taking care about the curation of the work I hope the work 'looks back', showing that it has been cared for. I hope my interactions with each artwork could become an added new force in the group matrix, a holding and containing one.

Group dynamics and the visual matrix

Although this is not an exhibition, there is a moment at the start that may echo the start of a therapy group, in the transition from social engagement, in this case art making and chatting, to the sense of sitting, looking, and waiting, to disengage socially perhaps, and get in touch with one's own self. This period holds a potential feeling of regression for group members and in the difficulty an idea of a leader is searched for, for answers. I am seen to move into an actively responsible role through my interactions and direct choices made for each artwork, but I do not make art, so as the group moves into the viewing there is an absence of my 'visual voice' in the group exhibition, which can create in me a feeling of impotence. There is an importance of this transitional space between one stage and another, where, as Yanagi describes it, we are 'lending an ear to what the object has to say' (2019: 281). This space may be anxiety provoking; the work may be 'likened to a mirror that passively reflects whatever is before it' (2019: 282) where the differences between works serve as a visual version of the differences between members. Often within a group, members will search at first for things that tie them together, possibly to strengthen the group; here, this can become like a necessity, something that may have informed the hanging and therefore informs the viewing.

We are also in a place of not knowing; in sitting being seen to be doing 'nothing' there may be an unspoken wish that I understand what is being looked at. The fantasy that as the therapist I can give meaning, with these expectations possibly heightened because of my directive action of curating and therefore also creating the potential for a further sense of disillusionment. This potential for the art to hold the feelings of anger, envy, hostility, and to be used expressively this way within the group is generally avoided. This may be for fear of any negative or hostile feelings coming to the surface and where a therapist may collude with the aim to create an experience of positivity by denying there is a space for difficult feelings (Dudley, 2012; Hinshelwood, 1987).

Filipovic suggests that an exhibition isn't only the sum of its artworks but also 'the relationships created between them, the dramaturgy around them, and the discourse that frames them' (2013: 75). This brings to mind the spaces each inhabits and the connections between the artworks. As works are recognised between members, and their internalised feelings around one another, there is a new potential for being seen and somehow known. In addition, works are sometimes admired, and this can be a boost to a fragile ego and will become part of a member's experience of the group. If the viewing is perceived to be aiming towards a supportive acceptance of one another through their art making, it can equally be interpreted to work as a kind of camouflage, where one could ask the question: What is not being said/seen? It is worth remembering that each member has chosen their own work, further selectively editing our process even before the viewing.

Berger (1972) suggests that paintings are objects of silence and stillness. He describes how an image can be affected by what it is seen besides and how words may change or inform how an image is perceived. This idea that until words are used, an artwork is silent, suggests to me it is the language itself that affects the viewing and, as Levens asks, 'What layers of background associations lie behind *each word for each individual* and simultaneously for the group in attempting to find shared meanings?' (2010: 18, italics mine). I would add here, what background associations relating to each artwork for each individual, and simultaneously within the group showing, lie behind each word spoken, each word heard, each work seen.

I wonder how the silence that begins each viewing is experienced and if this transition into looking is also a movement towards this idea of 'force and desire and intent' as described by Elkins earlier. What then does the speaking do in terms of looking together, if not a desire to alleviate the tension experienced in silence?

Conclusion

I have set out to think about why I curate the work in this group and what meanings it may have for members; between themselves and their artwork, each other, and the relationship to myself as therapist. I have thought about the effect of my own curatorial influences and how looking for one's artwork as placed or exhibited by another may provoke many responses, such as gratitude, feeling looked after, or feeling displaced or misplaced. My understanding of how artworks may be placed, and that the places may import messages unconsciously between members and myself, has meant that I have had to question further my physical interaction with the artworks. With each placing of each artwork in response to its colour, size, or mark, there has also been a group member and their relationship to myself attached, giving meaning that may be deeply connected to their own personal sense of self; from feeling seen as a young child, to being loved, wanted, admired, protected, or neglected, that has carried on to late adulthood. As material for the transference, the handling of artwork has potential for further exploration, but it has been my focus to think about the viewing with an exploration of my own curatorial role within the studio-based model of this particular group. I do feel that I took pleasure in these viewings, as a chance to interact with the artworks and provide care and respect for the work, with the hope that it was felt deeply and internalised by members. I consider they have been a way for me to provide group feedback, to almost rearrange how we as a group are progressing, and to create memories that shape the group culture.

References

Berger, J. (1972) *Ways of Seeing*. London, Penguin Books.
Dudley, J. (2012) The Art Psychotherapy Median Group. *Group Analysis*, 45(3): 325–338.
Elkins, J. (1996) *The Object Stares Back: On the Nature of Seeing*. New York, Harvest.

Filipovic, E. (2013) What is an Exhibition? In: Hoffmann, J. (ed.), *Ten Fundamental Questions of Curating*. Milan, Mousse Publishing.

Henley, D. (1992) Aesthetics in Art Therapy: Theory into Practice. *The Arts in Psychotherapy,* 19(3): 153–161.

Hinshelwood, R. (1987) *What Happens in Groups*. London, Free Association Press.

Levens, M. (2010) *Are Words Important in Group Analysis? An Exploration of the Consequences of Verbal Articulation*. MSc Dissertation, Birkbeck College, University of London.

Reagan, L. H. (2017) *Translating Principles from Art Curating to Art Therapy Practice: A Grounded Theory Research Study*. Doctoral dissertation, Mount Mary University.

Stacey, R. D. (2001) Complexity and the Group Matrix. *Group Analysis*, 34(2): 221–239.

Yanagi, S. (2019) *The Beauty of Everyday Things*. London, Penguin Classics.

16 Exploring experiences of exhibiting artwork from a therapeutic art studio for refugees and asylum seekers

Jon Martyn

This chapter seeks to continue a line of enquiry which began with 'Can Exhibiting Art Works from Therapy be Considered a Therapeutic Process?' (Martyn 2019). That article sought to unpack some of the contentious aspects of exhibiting artwork made in therapy and presented the approach developed at the New Art Studio (NAS), a therapeutic art studio for asylum seekers and refugees. While theorising and articulating this approach helped to conceptualise and ground my practice, the piece felt incomplete without the voice of the group members. In this chapter I hope to provide further understanding of the topic through interviews with six group members. Before coming to these I provide some aspects of the context through looking at some ideas about exhibiting, the studio itself, and the nature of asylum.

The therapeutic potential of exhibiting

Thompson (2009) suggests that the gallery can be seen as a potential space where an artist is able to explore and play with their relationship to society. The gallery offers opportunities for the artist to experiment with how they would like to be seen by others. Through exhibitions the gallery offers the opportunity for an artist to have their creations seen, discussed, and sold. And the private view gives opportunity for the artist to meet the public in a particular way – through a mutual interest in art.

While the exhibition offers experiences that go beyond what can be offered by a therapeutic environment, they are not able to offer therapeutic containment. The gallery is clearly distinct from therapeutic environments as it foregrounds the aesthetic and places an emphasis on a certain way of valuing art, most acutely experienced through the pricing and sales of art. More overtly than the therapeutic space, the gallery is open to market-driven forces and public curiosity. At its worst, the market is synonymous with exploitation and public curiosity can tip into voyeurism. Such experiences may be psychologically damaging and can lead to the artist feeling (further) objectified, exploited, devalued, and marginalised.

Yet exhibitions also have the potential to be political acts which challenge hegemony and give the public the opportunity to engage with social injustice and inequality. The exhibition can be seen as part of art therapy's long relationship with radical psychologies, which seek to challenge and change society (for example, the therapeutic

DOI: 10.4324/9781003095606-20

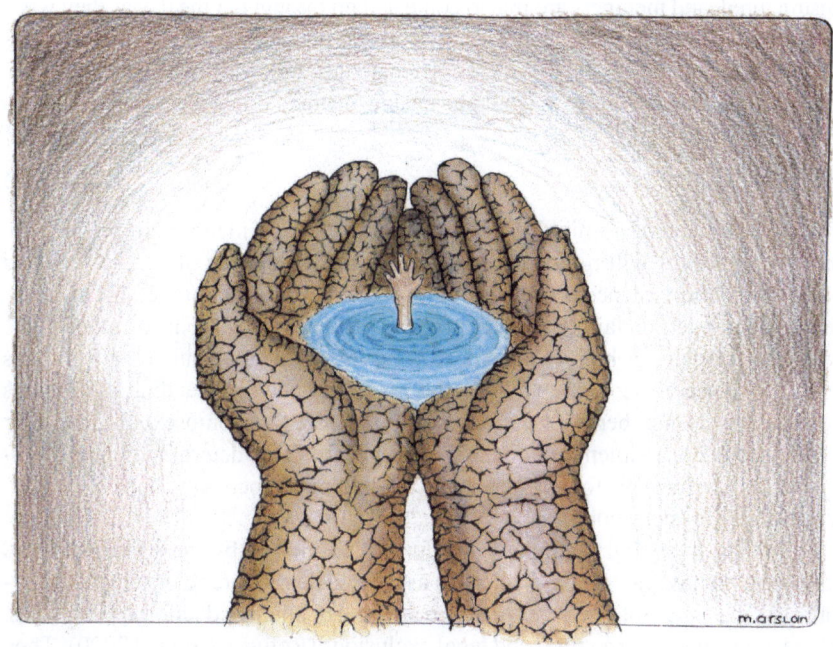

Figure 16.1 'Loneliness' by Mehmet Arslan.

community movement, antipsychiatry, Studio Upstairs,[1] and social action art therapy). Here, the exhibition offers the exhibitor an opportunity to step away from a marginalised and dehumanised position and be given the esteemed status of an artist. Perhaps, related to this is the potential for artworks to communicate in emotive and personal ways, which may provoke an intimate connection with the public (Potash et al. 2013). An exhibition can be transformative for both artists and the public.

The new art studio

NAS is a non-profit organisation for asylum seekers and refugees co-founded by art therapists Tania Kaczynski and myself in 2015. It is a therapeutic art studio, modelled on the Studio Upstairs, which sees exhibiting as a central part of its ethos. NAS is open one day a week for six hours. Its mixed-gender adult membership is predominantly from North Africa and Western Asia. The group is best described as a slow-open group, with members able to stay for as long as they wish; many staying in the group for years. In regard to the British legal system members will be at different stages of this lengthy, arduous, and humiliating process; with some seeking asylum, some having been granted the precarious 'right to remain', and some having British citizenship.

Aside from 'talking time', a thirty-minute section at the end of the day, the day is unstructured, and members are free to come and go throughout the day as they wish. They are encouraged to develop their own artistic practice as well as their relationships with the therapists and their peers. Art materials, food, drinks, and travel money are provided; and the majority would be unable to attend if this were not the case.

Asylum

The asylum seeker is a highly denigrated and excluded identity. To begin with, the asylum seeker will be forced into exile as a consequence of state-sanctioned persecution and violence. For some, simply being of the 'wrong' ethnic identity, sexuality, gender, or faith is enough to be at risk of persecution; for others, it is what they say, do, or believe. The need for political asylum can come from acts which may seem inconsequential to the reader – such as attending a women's demo, being a member of a political party, writing pro-homosexual graffiti, or wishing to leave a violent relationship. These acts of self-determination and self-protection can have profound consequences, leading the person to become a politicised target for persecution.

Following their flight, the person is further politicised by the so-called 'host' country, who now categorise them as an asylum seeker, migrant, or refugee. 'Asylum seeker', 'migrant', and 'refugee' are unwanted, alien, and enforced identities, which are subject to structural and legal exclusions (Refugee Council 2020). They are dehumanised identities, denigrated by the political establishment, and the right-wing press whose rhetoric enables far-right violence (Fekete 2018). They are severed identities; cut off from their language, family, culture, faith, and soil. Life in the UK is very difficult; the asylum seeker is prohibited from working, forced to depend on state support, and subject to a demonstrably racialised system of detention and deportation (Turnbull & Hasselberg 2017). The asylum seeker lives in a state of prolonged precarity, often in inadequate and unstable housing, while facing a lengthy and often retraumatising legal case before political asylum is granted. To compound this, the stability of asylum is increasingly fragile. In recent years, the UK government's 'Hostile Environment' policies, instigated by Theresa May whilst Home Secretary, have led to migrants being denied essential healthcare and, in some cases, having the legal protection of asylum and even their citizenship being revoked. As a consequence of state violence at home and the continued oppression and denigration in the UK, many prefer to stay within the safety of their own communities or in isolation.

In recognition of these multiple hostilities, NAS is run as a communal and supportive space. In addition to what NAS provides, members bring their own food to share and support each other, both emotionally and through their creative endeavours. In trying to describe this environment I am reminded of the term 'everyday communism', which David Greaber describes as: 'the raw material of sociality, a recognition of our ultimate interdependence that is the ultimate substance of social peace' (2011: 99). It is an environment where relations are not so concerned with reciprocity – the group has a distinct sense of generosity, solidarity, and

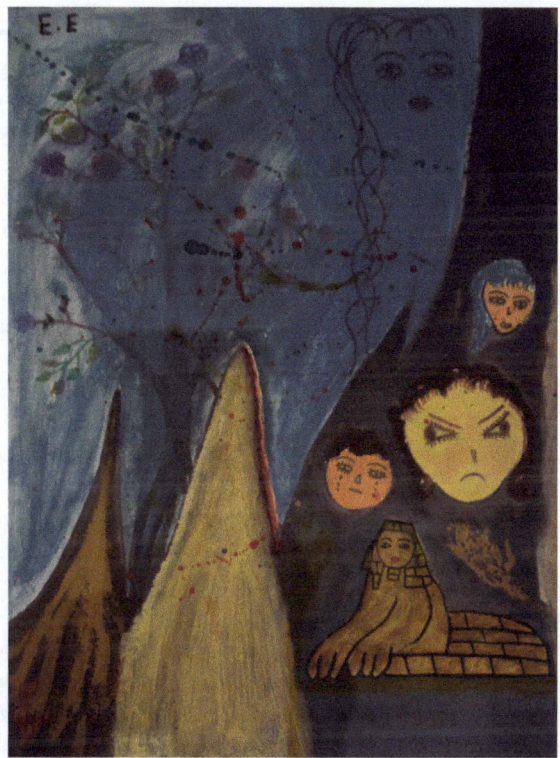

Figure 16.2 'Untitled' by E.E.

cooperation – but one where resources are pooled together to be shared. In the use of this phrase, I do not intend to idealise the space; there are certainly times when resources are not shared, and relations enter into disharmony, but these moments stand out as somewhat counter to the group's pervading culture. While this atmosphere of cooperation is certainly encouraged by its facilitators, there is a strong sense that it is co-created and sustained by the group's membership, an indication of an enduring desire for peace.

Exhibiting is firmly part of the studio's culture and, since its formation, members have wanted to exhibit, sell, and, when legally possible, receive money from their artwork. NAS sees the exhibition as an opportunity for the members to engage with the public and in turn, society. The exhibition takes time to set up and is facilitated to be a collaborative process, with members encouraged to participate in all aspects of the exhibitions, from selection, framing, naming, hanging, curating, and being part of the private view. Opportunity is given for members to speak at these events if they wish. Many members choose to exhibit under pseudonyms, and some choose not to exhibit at all. Exhibitions are not without difficulties and the therapeutic space is used to contain such experiences.

The interviews

Interviews were conducted in October 2020, fourteen months after leaving my role as co-facilitator. Prior to meeting, the six interviewees were given a series of open questions, which asked them to consider their experiences of exhibiting. These covered their difficulties, the selling of artwork, exhibiting as part of a group, and if they thought exhibiting could be therapeutic. Interviews were held individually and consisted of recorded conversations conducted in English, which were subsequently transcribed. One interviewee (Mr E) responded in writing; his response had been translated into English by his son.

I conducted an interview with co-founder Tania, the lead art therapist at the studio, whose thoughts set the scene for the members' comments that follow.

> *There's something life affirming about having an exhibition. A lot of difficulty in mental health is feeling that you are not being seen or understood by other people. So a feeling that you are being seen, understood and accepted by other people is really therapeutic. Most [members] live in an invisible place in society. It is particularly poignant to have a picture on the wall for the public to see. Art is a way of communicating with people you may never meet. It's a way of telling your story without standing in front of a person and telling your story. In some way it is a dialogue with the world.*
>
> *Exhibiting can be difficult, anxiety provoking. For the members, it's really rare to be in a public space when all eyes are on them. The members of the studio can meet the public as artists. That's quite refreshing when your identity is that of an asylum seeker, which often has quite negative associations. It is so different to be asked about the artwork, someone might ask you about red; "what does red mean to you?". It's a different type of attention, and talking about a different part of themselves. Sometimes you can literally see people get taller, as they speak with people, as they start owning their space, and owning the interest that someone else is giving them.*
>
> *To me money isn't a dirty word. There's nothing shameful about wanting money or getting money. It's not even the money so much, as somebody wants it. Somebody would like to take that home and have it in their sitting room. It makes you feel more integrated in the world. The weeks that follow an exhibition people have a lot of ideas, they want to paint more. It spurs them on. Quite soon people are asking when our next show will be.*

The following are comments from the transcribed interviews with the members. They have been ordered into themes and quotes have been chosen that add volition to the points. The monikers Mr A, Ms B, etc. follow the order in which I conducted the interviews.

All interviewees commented on a sense of unity that the setting up and curation of pictures brings, with it being described as a 'celebration' by Ms B. Of this, Mr C said, "I remember all of us, we were deciding pictures, and deciding which pictures go on which wall . . . and we were sharing that proud feeling". He goes on to describe the collaborative aspect of curation "finding which picture fits next to each other. Seeing how pictures fit together. Which colours fit well together. Deciding how to show them in the best possible way. Sharing the proudness together. It is really important". Ms F said "Build confidence and self esteem and believe in yourself. And go into public, step forward. That's it. All the way positive".

Speaking of his difficulty as an asylum seeker, Mr A said that exhibiting gave him a distinct sense of purpose "When you do not have your language, not have your home, you ask yourself – what am I living for? When you leave your country you lose hope. Lose your goals. I ask what am I living for?" Mr A saw art making and exhibiting as a new start "It is like I am born again. I never have a goal to paint or draw. I build myself as an artist. Exhibition gives me a challenge, and I need a challenge". He went on to describe exhibiting as a way of saying "I am here".

Mr E spoke positively of his experience at a private view.

> This experience taught me that you feel more confident in a group exhibition especially if you have a language barrier. This is important to gather artists, artworks and people. Artists meet new artists, people meet new ideas and opinions. It makes everyone excited and happy.

Mr E spoke of watching people respond to his artwork.

> [art] directs a mirror to people to show them their reality and truth. In this case, making the problems visible and warning people makes me excited and gives me happiness. I have seen people at the exhibition searching for meaning in my cartoons and their excitement as they find one, which made me happy.

Mr C explored how exhibiting helped him with language barriers.

> If we can't speak, we don't need to speak, the artwork is there and we share something . . . my artwork is describing itself. You don't need words to understand something, you can look and understand. You don't need to understand or feel the same thing, we can understand or interact in different ways, and it's totally ok. Because art is that.

Half the participants spoke of their difficulties in public. Mr A described a change that occurred with successive exhibitions:

> First time you feel stressed. But after you feel better and better. After my experiences you hide, but you need to be seen as a person. But you feel stressed, why am I feeling this? When you start again, it is very strange and very stressful, but it helps you after. It is one time, it's ok, its ok, it's ok, you are safe. Step by step. This helped me. Exhibiting helped me to overcome, I was in a position to overcome fear.

Similarly, Ms F said that she has "Too many difficulties" in public. Yet during exhibitions she has "No anxiety, because you help me. No pressure on me. I haven't got any anxiety because you [the therapists] do that. I haven't got any pressure on me".

Ms B explored mixed feelings about the artwork she exhibits:

> Do you really want to share this information with the people? What you share but what you don't share – so it's a confusing feeling when you exhibit your work. You want to share, but will they understand. You have a problem with immigration, but do you want to share this? Or share problems in your life? Do you want people to know you've been detained? Do you want people to know about domestic violence? I would like the people to know, but not know it has happened to me.

She acknowledged that she was new to exhibiting and hoped that this dilemma would improve with further experience.

Ms B also described negative experiences of exhibiting, describing her ambition to sell artwork and converse with the public. "Sometimes the exhibition does not bring good things. Some people sell works, sometimes people don't. So I think that my work is bad . . . I felt my pictures were ignored". She felt there was inequality in the way exhibitions were curated and promoted, with some members having more artworks than others and with promotional material focusing on a limited number of artworks. While she thought exhibiting could be therapeutic, she felt that the sales of artwork undermined this. "If you think about why I didn't sell, then [I feel] the opposite of happy, it is not great". Ms B added, "I do not want the studio to stop selling stuff, because it helps people". Ms D felt similarly to Ms B when I asked her if exhibiting was therapeutic, she replied, "Therapeutic? I don't think so. It's all about money! I mean it's most about money. Money becomes the biggest thing. Definitely". I asked her if the exhibition would be better without sales. "No one would put their artwork in. Everything is for money in this world. Studio is not about money, but the gallery is all about money". Both Ms B and Ms D plan to exhibit again, with Ms D emphasising her strong connections with the studio members, and Ms B considering how the group and facilitators might be able to support her with her difficulties.

Four interviewees had all sold artwork, and their view of sales was positive. Mr A, whose migration had forced him to be separated from his family said, "I put my soul into my picture. They are my feelings. But they are also money to see my family. When I fly to my family, to my wife, this is my price for my freedom to see them". Mr C said,

> I sold artwork and it was quite good. Selling is good for everyone. Especially if you are low income, almost nothing you are getting. It is not only about money: people want to see your artwork in their home, and they are paying money for this. It is something that can feel really good.

Ms F said,

> One of my artworks I wanted to throw out. My feeling was that it was not
> very good. But someone at an exhibition wanted to buy it. Before I didn't
> have any confidence in my paintings. But here, in exhibition, I understand
> that any piece of art is very important, it doesn't matter how I draw it, it is my
> feelings, I should keep it. I should respect my painting. If I respect my art,
> everyone can feel that.

Three interviewees explored how exhibitions give them an opportunity to learn
about British culture. Ms B said the exhibition can "tell me what the English public like – every country has their own taste. I would like to learn how the public
taste pictures". Ms D said,

> You can show your artwork, they can come see, give you comments about
> your work. And you know what is the weakness or power of your artwork.
> So that you can improve. It is a motivation to do better painting in the future.

Mr E saw the exhibition as an opportunity to learn about cultural differences in
the UK. "I have learned the things I need to consider when creating an exhibition.
I have learned that exhibiting style in England is really different from Turkey".

Mr A sees the exhibiting as an opportunity for the public to learn "Refugees
need the opportunity to share their experiences, as they can contribute to society.
Refugees can be stronger than others". Similarly, Mr E saw exhibitions as a place
for healing for both artists and the public.

> Art is a work that repairs spirits and psychology. In addition to being a heal-
> ing medicine of art, it is a food that prevents disease from the very beginning,
> it is the food of the soul and humanity. If the world will reach peace, friend-
> ship, justice and freedom, it can only achieve this through art.

Discussion

The excerpts from these interviews speak of the sometimes-conflicted potential
of exhibitions. They illustrate how an exhibition can offer the opportunity to
improve a sense of oneself by engaging with the public and how the process
of setting up an exhibition can be a collaborative and cohesive experience, one
which offers opportunity for celebration. All interviewees indicated a desire to
meet and communicate with the public and valued the opportunity to do this as
a group. There were indications that members were using exhibitions to experiment with the way they are seen. For example, with Ms B still exploring how
she'd like to be seen by the public and Mr A describing his artistic identity as
a new life. The opportunity to exhibit was challenging, but as explained by
Mr A and Ms F, when one feels held by the group, difficulties can diminish with
successive exhibitions.

Also highlighted is a contrast between the studio space and the gallery. It is evident that the curation, promotion, and sales of artwork bring competitiveness, which can leave artists feeling ignored and undervalued – particularly when the artist does not sell. While exhibitions may disturb the sense of the studio's communality in this way, there are indications that this was neither unbearable nor unrepairable. The interviewees' continued connection with the NAS indicates that the emotional difficulties provoked by exhibitions can be held and worked through in the therapeutic art studio. Both Ms B and Ms D wished to exhibit again, and Ms D wanted to emphasise the kinship she felt in the studio. Just as the therapeutic space offers opportunity to contain difficult experiences, the interview offered Ms B the opportunity to articulate her discontent and led her to consider sharing this with NAS therapists and peers. While sales remain a somewhat contentious issue, it is clear that all interviewees wanted the opportunity to sell and receive income from their artwork. To me, this suggests that sales, and their temporary relief from poverty, are seen as more important than the psychological cost of feeling ignored.

Selling art evidently offers psychological gains with Ms F indicating that the sale of an artwork gave her confidence. Her statement, "If I respect my art, everyone can feel that", suggests a change in her which led to a change in the way she is perceived by others. Mr C's reference to an artwork being in someone's home resonates with Tania's belief that sales lead the artist to feeling more integrated with the world. Sales were emotively explored by Mr A – the money gave him the opportunity to see his family, which he equated to freedom.

The private view presents opportunities to meet the public in ways that are, perhaps, unique. Mr C and Mr E both describe experiences as exhibiting artists which transcend language barriers, pointing to the potential of art to form connections beyond spoken language. Mr E's statement 'artist's meet other artists' indicates a levelling out of status, with members and the public standing together, sharing a mutual appreciation of the art, forming relationships, and sharing ideas. Ms B, Ms D, and Mr E shared their interest in learning about public taste, aesthetics, and curation, and there is an indication that the exhibition presents an opportunity for the artists to better understand the public. This is something particularly pertinent for those living in the margins of a foreign and often hostile society.

If the gallery is to be considered a potential space, then we must see it as an opportunity for the public to be changed by the artists. Exhibiting offers the opportunity for the public not only to learn from but stand with and connect to the artists in a highly personal way. This point relates to the notion of cultural integration, an idea that often emphasises the migrant's need to adapt to the host culture. Yet, as Mr A justly points out, we 'the hosts' have much to gain if we are open to being changed by the migrant. Echoing Graeber (2011), Mr E indicates that art offers us opportunity for peace, friendship, justice, and freedom. These can only be achieved if we are willing to consider our interdependence by learning from and standing with those who are denigrated and excluded.

Note

1   Therapeutic art studio established in 1988 on the principles of R.D. Laing and the Philadelphia Association.

References

Fekete, E. (2018) *Europe's fault lines: Racism and the rise of the right*. London, Verso Books.

Graeber, D. (2011) *Debt: The first, 5000 years*. Brooklyn, Melville House Publishing.

Martyn, J. (2019) Can exhibiting art works from therapy be considered a therapeutic process? *ATOL: Art Therapy Online, 10*(1). Available at: https://journals.gold.ac.uk/index.php/atol/article/view/548/pdf.

Potash, J.S., Ho, R.T.H., Chick, J.K.Y. and Yeung, F.A. (2013) Viewing and engaging in an art therapy exhibit by people living with mental illness: Implications for empathy and social change. *Public Health, 127*(8): 735–744.

Refugee Council (2020) *The Truth About Asylum – Refugee Council*. [online] Available at: <https://refugeecouncil.org.uk/information/refugee-asylum-facts/the-truth-about-asylum/> [Accessed 17 November 2020].

Thompson, G. (2009) Artistic sensibility in the studio and gallery model: Revisiting process and product. *Art Therapy, Journal of the American Art Therapy Association, 26*(4): 159–166.

Turnbull, S. and Hasselberg, I. (2017) From prison to detention: The carceral trajectories of foreign-national prisoners in the United Kingdom. *Punishment & Society, 19*(2): 135–154.

17 Private to public

Exhibition in art therapy

Mary Andrus

Your silence will not protect you.

– Audre Lorde

Art therapy provides an opportunity to amplify marginalised voices, raise awareness, expand critical consciousness, and move beyond private spaces into the public to impact social perceptions and create change. Moving stories and artwork
out of traditionally private spaces into the public creates the potential for change
in the client, for the public who are witnesses to the art and story, and for the collective group who are sharing their stories (Andrus, 2019). There is therapeutic
value in creating spaces to impact interpersonal, intrapersonal, and greater societal change. Lorde (1992), a feminist writer and activist, aptly articulated this
sentiment in the aforementioned quote.

Art therapy in the US emerged from Western ideas with psychoanalytic and
psychodynamic roots, resulting in a field with a tradition of dichotomous thinking.
The binary thinking in art therapy of 'art psychotherapy' versus 'art as therapy',
or the 'clinical' versus 'studio' duality, is not representative of everyday practice
of art therapy (Potash et al., 2016). In recent years, scholars have noted a lack
of social justice theory integrated into art therapy practices (Kaplan & Sajnani,
2012; Talwar, 2019). As a result, art therapists have been slow to move towards
an integration of more socially conscious practices designed to help equalise the
power differential in treatment.

This chapter includes (a) a rationale for shifting the practice of art therapy to
focus on expanding connections with communities, (b) an examination of the
potential impact of moving therapeutic artwork into the public as a part of treatment, and (c) examples to outline ways to shift art therapy practices. I will discuss
a case example of creating a film with a client in private practice who experienced
a trauma and then reintegration once she moved her story into the public. Also,
I will share outcomes from a community of women who participated in the Bearing Witness exhibitions of artwork about pregnancy loss, infertility, and stillbirth
(Andrus, 2019). Moving their private pain into a public exhibition and creation of
a film (Andrus, 2017) about their stories led to therapeutic growth that they could
not have accomplished on their own.

DOI: 10.4324/9781003095606-21

Social, political, and cultural issues

A feminist, narrative, and social constructionist approach can help clients identify their story and deconstruct how it has been situated via their social location (Hogan, 1997). Within this framework, the therapist is aware of their power and privilege in the relationship (hooks, 2015). A social constructionist approach moves away from an emphasis on pathology or dysfunction looking at ways to build resilience (Riley, 1997; Springham, 2016). As clients identify their story and share it with the therapist, the story is re-storied (White & Epston, 1990). Part of the work is moving the story out of the private into another space, such as a studio exhibiting space, to de-centre the therapist as the objective expert (Payne, 2006; Andrus, 2019).

Many art therapists value the art created by unseen populations, using exhibition to raise awareness, address stigma, reduce isolation, and increase empathy of witnesses through public exhibition (Ho et al., 2017; Lu & Yuen, 2012; Koh & Shrimpton, 2014; DeLucia, 2016). Concerns of exploitation are legitimate for non-art therapists who are not trained or required to abide by the same ethical principles as art therapists when exhibiting artwork to promote awareness of social issues (Davis, 2017). Scholars have begun examining the intersection of art therapy in museums (Salom, 2011; Rochford, 2017; Potash, 2016), where the art serves as a stimulus for dialogue and reflection.

People seek therapy when their lived reality does not match the dominant discourse (White & Epston, 1990). Navigating life where this is not in alignment can be isolating and feel oppressive. When we connect our stories to one another, we feel a sense of belonging and understanding (Brown, 2012). In order for liberation to occur within oppressed groups of people, they must move through phases of understanding that lead towards transformation (Friere, 2000).

The storied narrative that emerges from the collective creates a space to challenge truths that have been socially constructed. Women in society have been socialised to stay silent and ascribe to the powerful's definition of their reality (hooks, 2015). They are bound by patriarchy and learn that their voice is not valued in society. Elthaway (2019) suggests that when women come together, share their experiences, challenge patriarchy, they embrace their personal power to push against the dominant narrative. She envisions a world where girls and women use their power to destroy their predators. She wrote: 'We are volcanos, when we women offer our experience as our truth, as human truth, all the maps change' (2019: 22).

In society, we tend to privilege stories and voices of some groups over others, which is an epistemic injustice (Fricker, 2007). For example, women who become pregnant are instructed to keep it private until after they reach twelve weeks (Bergbom et al., 2017). This attunement to power brings up a variety of questions for disempowered populations. When women are faced with the burden of staying silent in their losses, what message are we sending? Why must they have to protect others from their pain? How does this social, cultural practice of protection actually cause harm to the woman and create a cycle of guilt, shame, and fear?

Trauma

Treatment of trauma builds through stages that start by developing strategies for self-regulation and attunement, then working through the story by telling the story in sequence, retelling it, and then moving into reintegration (Shapiro, 2012; Herman, 2019). Research that examines the neurological impact of trauma shows that sensory information encodes in the amygdala and the Broca's area, or speech centre, turns off when the fight, flight, freeze impulse takes over (van der Kolk, 2014; Siegel, 2010; Cozolino, 2010). There is significant healing that comes from telling, retelling, and witnessing the story being told (Gantt & Tinnin, 2007; Chapman, 2014; Cohen & Orr, 2015). I posit that the actual resolution of trauma occurs when the story is moved out of the private, into the public and is affirmed by a group of empathic public witnesses. Until this is facilitated and experienced by the person who experienced the trauma, they may not be able to see themselves as separate from the experience.

When coordinating an exhibition that represents pain, trauma, or difficult life experiences, the display of the artwork should be curated with care. The exhibit should be presented in an emotionally supportive environment, where the impact of the show can create more awareness, empathy, and knowledge about the topic (Koh & Shrimpton, 2014). This helps the artists be seen, heard, and the viewers to come out with more understanding of mental health issues.

Case study

This is the story about a client that I worked with years ago. The details of her trauma experience are not important. They are not mine to tell you. They are hers. Little did we know that this work would transform our paths, creating such depth and resonance for growth. On our first meeting, she wheeled in a medium-sized black suitcase beside her and placed it next to the table. She averted eye contact, had a soft-spoken tone of voice and trouble finding words to describe her experiences.

Telling

My internal awareness acknowledged that we both were middle aged, able bodied, middle class, white women with privilege and means to move in and out of society with ease and comfort. We made some connections and then she looked at her suitcase. She pulled out a stack of drawings she had made on mat boards to process her experiences. One by one, she added them into a pile reaching at least one foot high on the table between us. This was the beginning of our journey.

Her experiences expanded beyond this small studio space in this urban community in the US and had reached lands far away with cross-cultural interactions that challenged her notion of safety. Her social location and visible white identity had allotted her freedoms that others were unable to access. Over time, we concluded that a series of traumatic instances, 'small t's' and 'big T's', left her in a state of inability to form words around her experiences, and post-traumatic stress had paralysed her functioning for years.

She controlled the pacing, with no pressure for her to have resolution or healing within a specified time frame. About two years or so in our work together, we started documenting her stories on video, I had a hunch that it would be important for her to have some of these stories reflected back to her.

Uncovering

There was power in her imagery that she could not comprehend on her own. When she shared her work with friends, they would have strong emotional reactions, but she did not allow herself to feel anything. She had been socialised to silence difficult feelings. In art therapy, she worked to access and identify her feelings, explore the narrative associated with each image, connecting the art to her felt experience.

One day she brought in an evocative image representing the moment in which her 'big T' trauma had occurred. I asked her to make three more pictures to explain this image, she came back with a stack of ten. We carefully looked at each image and processed them individually. She slowly read a written narrative aloud as she pointed to each drawing. She meticulously rendered the moment in time when her brain was encoded with sensory data and the Broca's area, or narrative memory, shut down. As she read the story associated with her imagery, she felt sick to her stomach. We realised that she had begun to externalise her story. She could choose when to look at it, noting that it was still hard to talk about it, but she felt proud for putting her story in the image rather than it living inside her mind every day.

Retelling

The next time we met, I taped the images to the wall in sequence, recorded her talking through each image (Figure 17.1) and telling the story again. It was hard, but she persisted. She spoke in a monotone voice and felt queasy when she talked. A few weeks later she asked if she could have another chance to tell the story, with just talking, *not reading her notes*. I recorded her retelling the story. This time, her affect changed, her voice had more emotional variation, a brightness appeared in her eyes, and when she was finished, she raised her hands in the air and expressed "YES!" She reflected that this was the first time that *she did not feel sick when talking about it*. We had captured transformative growth, it was powerful, the story was shifting from controlling her, to something she was able to see outside of herself.

With her permission, I presented her story in a short film I had made for a local conference. She did not attend, but admittedly was unable to sit and watch the film in its entirety. The audience participants were moved by her artwork and story and wanted to ask her questions about it. She was happy to hear it was of interest to people but was not fully able to understand why. I was keenly aware of the power differential and how it was her story to share.

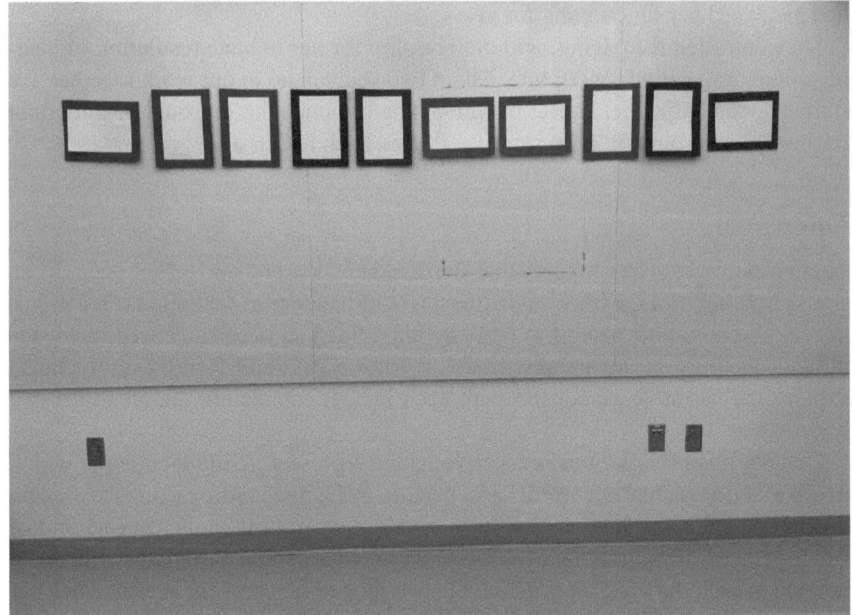

Figure 17.1 The eye series (recreation of original image).

Witnessing

A year later, an Art Therapy Symposium was upcoming in the neighbouring state, and I proposed to her that we tell the story together. I could present the film; she could be there to watch it and then the audience could ask her questions directly. She agreed, reflected that she didn't need it for herself, but she'd do it if it would help the field of art therapy. She had not fully sat down and watched the film at this point. Her partner had her watch it prior to attending the Symposium, which she was hesitant to do. She felt detached from the story, saw the film as my 'project', not something that we were co-constructing together.

After we co-presented her story publicly, she reflected that she thought that telling her story might help others but realised that it actually did help her grow. A few months later she expressed a renewed interest in the film, amending, adding, making suggestions for edits. The film became my response art to her story, but it also became our story as we co-constructed meaning for her from her experience. She then shared the film with her with parents and felt proud of her story for the first time.

Reflecting

In writing this chapter, I grappled with how to write and still preserve the integrity of her story. I purposely omitted details that would identify her and reconnected with her and her partner when composing this chapter. We spoke specifically about what was most helpful to them in moving her story out of the private into the public. Presenting publicly was a big step for her. She had not left the state in over ten years and cried throughout the drive from her home to the Symposium. She was worried and nervous of facing the unknown of presenting. Once other people saw it, acknowledged it, accepted it, had questions about it, she was able to talk openly about it with others. She stated: "sharing the video gave me affirmative feedback that I had been taking positive steps towards recovery". Sharing the story with a public audience was pivotal to her reintegration. On the drive home her partner noticed, "there was no crying, her spirit was different, more confident, with no fear, whatever happened when she stood up in front of that group, there was a noticeable shift". She said, "I own this, I did this" (Personal communication August 1, 2020).

She moved from the dorsal frozen state into attuned state of engagement with the world. The compulsion to create or the need to continue telling the story was no longer there. Public sharing gave her the courage to share it with the people she wanted to understand the most, her family.

It was in her imaging, writing, telling, retelling, witnessing, reflecting, sharing, and resharing her story that she was able to find meaning. Trauma was transformed by finding meaning in the story, using the story to empower others, to give her purpose, and to help her define who she was, separate from the traumatic experiences. The film became a container, a reflection of her story, and an important part of her healing. It leaves me wondering if I had not captured her story on film and shared it publicly, would she have had such transformative growth? Why do we work so hard to protect our clients' stories? This work inspired me to begin my doctorate in art therapy to investigate the intersection of public and private in art therapy.

Reauthoring our collective stories

When entering the last year of my doctoral studies, I reached out to an art therapist colleague on the West Coast who had coordinated two art exhibitions four years prior, featuring artwork from women who experienced miscarriage, repeated infertility, or stillbirth. I reached out to her and asked if she thought the artists from her show might be interested in being a part of a research project in an attempt to retrospectively understand if it was helpful to have their work on display in a public exhibition.

I designed a phenomenological, arts-based research study that examined the impact of sharing publicly. From the thirty artists who were in the show, half agreed to participate in my study. The project was approved by Mount Mary University's institutional review board. I communicated to the artist participants that I was going to be creating a film about their art and stories. I collected their artwork and the written artist statements from the artists. I collected consent forms as it related to the level of involvement with the project; some artists just submitted work to be included in a film about their experience, others were interviewed as a group or individually.

Permutations of sharing

Prior to sharing their art, the women felt isolated, unsupported, hidden shame and guilt, and that their loss was unreal (Andrus, 2019). Many had experienced unhelpful comments from people in their lives. All those who were interviewed said that they were afraid to share their stories. They were not only holding their own pain and grief, but they were also protecting others from their pain, realising for some, it was too much to bear.

Some described a cathartic release through the exhibitions. Several mentioned that the exhibition helped them to embrace their truth, others uncovered additional grief that they had not acknowledged. Many connected with things that were expressed in one another's artwork that they did not have the words for, they stated "I felt that way too". They found validation and acknowledgement that their loss was real. The art served as an outlet for them, and they found strength in the community of artist participants.

Women who experience miscarriage or repeated infertility bear an invisible burden of grief (Andrus, 2019). Prior to the exhibits they felt isolated, and after they felt affirmed. One of the artists shared that she was hesitant to share her art with people, fearing they might think she was weird. Another expressed isolation in her grief, stating that there was nothing out there for her when she was struggling with her losses. She posted her artwork images to a Flicker© site noting that it was affirming to her to see that a thousand people looked at her work online. Another artist shared that it was strange to feel so good to be a part of a show that was all about death and dying. There was a cathartic release that came from being in a supportive space with people who shared her experience and understood her grief. Another after seeing the first show (Figure 17.2) expressed interest in showing her art in the second show (Figure 17.3). This led her to have the courage to speak on a panel in front of hundreds of nurses at a conference about her losses. She shared that when she had her work in the show she was not 100% comfortable telling everyone about her story but putting the work in the shows gave her courage to participate in the research project.

A year later, I invited a group of the women from the research to present the film publicly at a conference. Three participants co-presented their stories. They reflected to me that having the film to contain their stories together was powerful, meaningful, and transformative for them. They were able to find strength in their collective voices and could see the benefit of sharing their stories with the larger community to raise critical consciousness about the experiences of women in society. They have since expressed interest in future public showings of the film so they can share it with their close family members, friends, and others to help them understand the pain, their losses and to honour the lives of their unborn babies.

Moving stories out of private spaces into the public is something that should be handled with care, ensuring you are not exploiting the people's stories and that they have ownership of the story, deciding where, when, and how it is told. From the women in this chapter, all of them consciously decided to move their story

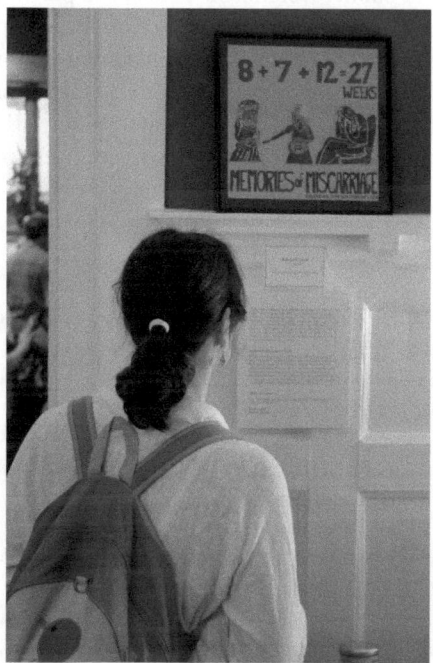

Figure 17.2 Bearing witness exhibit at the Peace House, May 2013.

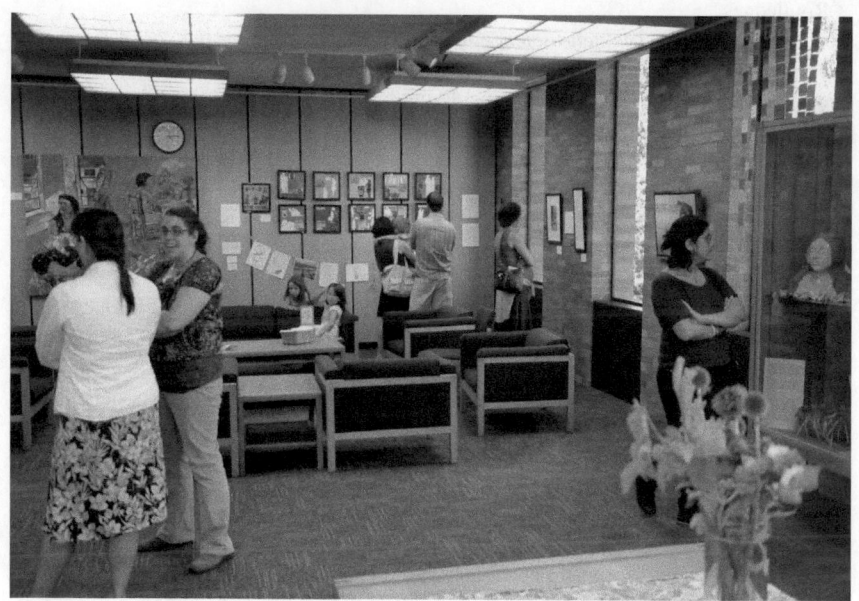

Figure 17.3 Bearing witness exhibit at Marylhurst University, June 2013.

and art from private to public, weighing the risks and potential benefits of taking action. There is collective power that comes out of bringing people together who have shared experiences to illuminate the connections that make us human and challenge the normative–non-normative dichotomy that exists in society. An art therapy studio exhibition space can be the container for this work. It is time for women to rise up, challenge patriarchy and misogyny, speak out, and unapologetically tell the stories of our lived experiences through our art.

References

Andrus, M. (Producer & Director) (2017). *Bearing witness film* [Doctoral research film]. Miwaukee, WI: Mount Mary University.

Andrus, M. (2019). Exhibition and film about infertility, miscarriage and stillbirth: Art therapy implications. *Art Therapy: Journal of the American Art Therapy Association*. 37(4): 169–176.

Bergbom, I., Modh, C., Lundgren, I., & Lindwall, L. (2017). First-time pregnant women's experiences of their body in early pregnancy. *Scandinavian Journal of Caring Sciences*. 31: 579–586

Brown, B. (2012). *Daring greatly: How the courage to be vulnerable transforms the way we love, parent and lead*. New York: Gotham Books.

Chapman, L. (2014). *Neurobiologically informed trauma therapy with children and adolescents: Understanding mechanisms of change*. New York: W.W. Norton & Company.

Cohen, J. L., & Orr, P. P. (2015). Film/video-based therapy and editing as process from a depth psychological perspective. In J. L. Cohen, J. L. Johnson, & P. P. Orr (Eds.), *Video and filmmaking as psychotherapy: Research and practice* (pp. 29–42). New York: Routledge.

Cozolino, L. (2010). *The neuroscience of psychotherapy: Healing the social brain* (2nd ed.). New York: W.W. Norton & Company.

Davis, T. (2017). Art therapy exhibitions: Exploitation or advocacy? *AMA Journal of Ethics, Images of Healing and Learning*. 19(1): 98–106.

DeLucia, J. (2016). Art therapy services to support veteran's transition to civilian life: The studio and the gallery. *Art Therapy: Journal of the American Art Therapy Association*. 33(1): 4–12.

Elthaway, M. (2019). *The seven necessary sins of women and girls*. Boston, MA: Beacon Press.

Fricker, M. (2007). *Epistemic injustice: Power and ethics of knowing. Hermeneutical injustice*. Oxford: Oxford Scholarship.

Friere, P. (2000). *Pedagogy of the oppressed*. New York: Bloomsbury Press.

Gantt, L., & Tinnin, L. W. (2007). Intensive trauma therapy of PTSD and dissociation: An outcome study. *Arts in Psychotherapy*. 34(1): 69–80.

Herman, J. (2019). *Group trauma treatment in early recovery: Promoting safety and self-care*. New York: The Guilford Press.

Ho, R., Potash, J., Ho, A., Ho, V., & Chen, E. (2017). Reducing mental illness stigma and fostering empathic citizenship: Community arts collaborative approach. *Social Work in Mental Health*. 15(4): 469–485.

Hogan, S. (1997). *Feminist approaches to art therapy*. New York: Routledge.

hooks, b. (2015). *Feminist theory: From margin to center*. New York: Routledge.

Kaplan, F., & Sajnani, N. (2012). The creative arts therapies and social justice: A conversation between the editors of this special issue. *The Arts in Psychotherapy.* 39(3): 165–167.

Koh, E., & Shrimpton, B. (2014). Art promoting mental health literacy and a positive attitude towards people with experience of mental illness. *International Journal of Social Psychiatry.* 60(2): 169–174.

Lorde, A. (1992). Quotations from Audre Lorde. *Off Our Backs.* 22(11): 3–23. Retrieved July 14, 2021, from www.jstor.org/stable/25775820.

Lu, L., & Yuen, F. (2012). Journey women: Art therapy in a decolonizing framework of practice. *The Arts in Psychotherapy.* 39(3): 192–200.

Payne, M. (2006). *Narrative therapy* (2nd ed.). London, England: Sage.

Potash, J. S. (2016). Response art: Using creative activity to deepen exhibit engagement. In E. M. Gokcigdem (Ed.), *Fostering empathy through museums* (pp. 77–91), Lanham, MD: Rowman & Littlefield.

Potash, J. S., Mann, S., Martinez, J., Roach, A., & Wallace, N. (2016). Spectrum of art therapy practice: Systemic literature review of art therapy. *Art Therapy: Journal of the American Art Therapy Association.* 33(3): 119–127.

Riley, S. (1997). Social constructionism: The narrative approach and clinical art therapy. *Art Therapy: Journal of the American Art Therapy Association.* 14(4): 282–284.

Rochford, J. S. (2017). Art therapy and art museum education: A visitor focused collaboration. *Art Therapy: Journal of the American Art Therapy Association.* 34(4): 209–214.

Salom, A. (2011). Reinventing the setting: Art therapy in museums. *The Arts in Psychotherapy.* 38(2): 81–85.

Shapiro, F. (2012). *Getting past your past: Take control of your life with self-help techniques from EMDR therapy.* New York: Rodale.

Siegel, D. (2010). *The developing mind: Toward a neurobiology of interpersonal experience.* New York: The Guilford Press.

Springham, N. (2016). Description as social construction in UK art therapy research. *International Journal of Art Therapy.* 21(3): 104–115.

Talwar, S. (2019). *Art therapy for social justice: Radical intersections.* New York: Routledge.

van der Kolk, B. (2014). *The body keeps the score: Brain, mind and body in the healing of trauma.* New York: Viking Penguin.

White, M., & Epston, D. (1990). *Narrative means to therapeutic ends.* New York: W.W. Norton & Company.

18 Making space

Art, the studio, and exhibition in homelessness services

Simon Richardson

London like other large cities has a deep-seated homelessness problem. Rough sleeping levels remain high while hidden homelessness (people 'sofa surfing' or living in squats or other insecure accommodation) reflects a lack of affordable housing. Services to tackle homelessness, mostly provided through the charitable or non-statutory sector, offer temporary accommodation and a range of support to help people stabilise their lives. I am going to describe studio art therapy sessions I ran in three different settings (a rolling shelter, an accommodation-based project, and a recovery college) within one such organisation. In doing so, I will focus on three key aspects: art, the studio, and exhibition and discuss the contribution of each to the creation of an art therapy process.

Achieving a coherent structure for studio art therapy in these services involved revisiting some fundamental ideas about practice. The core aim was to offer sessions in which people could engage in creative activity within an accessible and supportive environment. Yet none of the available theoretical models quite seemed to encompass this. Case and Dalley describe the 'studio-based open group' as the classic form of art therapy, but one that was 'the main way of working before training was available in the early 1970s' (2014: 151). Moon takes a more positive stance, suggesting studio art therapy is better understood as an 'art-based art therapy practice' (2002: 21). While this resonates more with the sessions I will describe, the term 'art-based' is not without complications (as I will discuss later). Meanwhile, homeless services frame activities (including art) as broadly educational, supporting learning or skills acquisition. While this is held to be person-centred and strengths-based it effectively maintains a notion of art as a set of practical techniques.

Thinking about art

The client's image is a central aspect of art therapy theory and practice. Case and Dalley describe it as mediating between the 'inner world and outer reality', containing symbolic material that can be worked on as part of the therapeutic relationship (2014: 105). This sets a psychoanalytically informed paradigm of the image in art therapy as a 'pictorial expression of inner experience' (2014: 86). I will refer to this henceforth as the standardised model. Intrinsic to this concept

DOI: 10.4324/9781003095606-22

of images is that they symbolise and have meaning. Mitchell discusses how this view of the image has evolved out of a centuries-old philosophical debate over the relationship between images and words, culminating in the modern pictorial image which he characterises as 'linguistic in its inner workings' (1987: 43). The standardised model is simply one example of this. However, revisiting this debate in the context of art therapy invites the question: Must art (the image) necessarily be symbolic (linguistic) to have therapeutic potential?

This links to a wider issue: that the standardised model has meant art therapists no longer consider 'What is art?' in their practice, creating a disconnect from the very thing that is nominally at its heart. Art theorists generally have found the question 'What is art?' far from straightforward. Carroll (1999), Hatt and Klonk (2006), and Warburton (2003) among others detail the problems arising from attempts to resolve it. 'Art' has come to be recognised as a contested term that resists a generic definition. Indeed the question, 'What is art?' effectively functions now as a paradox, being simultaneously a philosophical dead end but equally a trap into which the unwary can fall. Something of this has happened in art therapy: holding the standardised model to be 'What is art?' has made other uses of art, however therapeutic, theoretically problematic.

I have discussed earlier how art therapy mostly sidesteps this issue (Richardson, 2015). Even Moon, who describes her practice as 'art-based' and is open to making 'art' as expansive as possible, still effectively takes the term as settled (2002: 47). These kinds of inconsistencies show how art therapy struggles to account for art being therapeutic outside the standardised model. What is needed is to re-engage with the question of 'art' in art therapy. With this in mind I want to look at two distinct approaches to what art is – or can be. The first is Goodman's study of symbol systems in *Languages of Art* (1976), and the second is Gell's account of art as social interaction in *Art and Agency* (1998).

Density and repleteness

Goodman delineates two main kinds of symbol system: 'differentiated' *linguistic* systems (such as languages or texts) and 'dense' *nonlinguistic* systems (such as pictures or images). I will focus on two aspects of nonlinguistic systems, their being 'semantically dense' and 'relatively replete'. Mark making, to take one example, is *semantically dense* in that every mark (its length, weight, shade, or tone) is different. Marks can be made in an infinite number of ways and cannot be isolated as distinct characters, whereas in differentiated systems like alphabets each letter corresponds to a unique character. A picture or an image is *relatively replete* in that a greater number of its features are relevant to the determination of meaning. Goodman exemplifies this by comparing a drawing of Mount Fuji by Hokusai with an electrocardiogram (1976: 229). Both have an undulating black line on a white background. Yet while every aspect of Hokusai's drawing has potential significance (even the paper on which it is drawn) only one aspect of the line in the electrocardiogram matters.

Thinking about Goodman's ideas in relation to art therapy, any engagement with a surface (from blots, scribbles, or smudges through to a formal pictorial image) can have semantic potential. All works can then be approached with an openness to their communicative possibilities. Because a primary feature of non-linguistic systems is there being no invariant relation between a dense symbol like a mark and what it represents (as Gaiger (2008) and Mitchell (1986) discuss in considering Goodman's work) a whole range of variables can manifest throughout the creative process. Inherent in making and looking at an image therefore is participation in a particular kind of (nonlinguistic) symbolic interaction, involving attention to every aspect of the work.

Indexing agency

Gell sets out to challenge the very idea 'that (visual) art is 'like language' and that the relevant forms of semiosis are language-like' (1998: 14). He proposes thinking about an 'art object' (indeed any objects people make) as an index of agency. The term 'index' derives from the semiotics of C.S. Pierce and means a sign directly or causally related to its object; Gell cites Pierce's example of smoke being indexical of fire (1998: 13). An art object for Gell is an index of its maker and their agency, an outcome of their actions and intentions. 'Index' confers no innate value as 'art' on an object but enables Gell to focus on how it functions as a nexus of social relations, both from the position of 'agent' (affecting others) and 'patient' (affected by others). Sansi explains how Gell utilises the anthropological concept of the 'partible' or 'distributed person' in order to treat 'art objects' as persons or extensions of persons (2015: 11). Gell uses the work of Marcel Duchamp and Maori meeting houses to show how an individual artist's *oeuvre* or the collective production of a community can be understood as a 'distributed object' (1998: 235). People as 'social persons' are present not just in their physical bodies but in everything which evidences their existence, attributes, and agency (1998: 103). Art objects are not simply passive containers of meaning but, as extensions of people, active participants in social action.

Where does this leave us with thinking about art in art therapy? Goodman and Gell occupy very different theoretical positions, but what unites them is not seeing 'art' as a defined set of objects or practices. Goodman focuses on how symbol systems function but, as Mitchell (1986) discusses, makes no stipulations about when they should be used. He resets 'What is art?' to 'When is art?' putting the emphasis on what art does rather than what it is (1978: 70). Gell's ideas might seem almost heretical for art therapy where so much focus has been on symbolism. Yet art therapy is a relational practice, and his focus on the index as a nexus of relations suggests how the interactions around art making in studio art therapy can make it more than simply a diversionary or skills-based activity.

Studio art therapy

The structure for studio art therapy in the homelessness settings I will describe was that people had access to a social space in which all aspects of their presence in the session and engagement with the media were valued and worked with as potentially meaningful. The sessions were open to anyone and people could attend for as long as they felt able to be there. There was no formalised referral system or assessment process in place and consequently no therapeutic contract. For this reason I have not included any illustrations of work made, with pseudonyms used throughout.

I ran the sessions at different times between 2008 and 2018 as a volunteer. While this had the effect of differentiating me from staff in how I was perceived by clients, I was still required to carry a walkie-talkie and a panic alarm during sessions at the rolling shelter and accommodation-based project. In both these settings, I would provide staff on shift with a brief handover after the session. The 'studio' in all the settings was a multi-use room that had to be set out and tidied away each time, with a range of art materials including acrylic paint, charcoal, crayons, oil pastels, and coloured pencils made available. Work could either be left with me and stored in a portfolio or taken away after the session.

A rolling shelter

Rolling shelters (a service model no longer used) were short-stay assessment services where people found rough sleeping could be housed while more permanent accommodation was sought for them. The shelters shadowed street homeless populations and could relocate quickly to be close to hotspots. The shelter where I volunteered wanted art therapy to contribute to the process of engaging with clients, many of whom were still partly living on the street. Sessions were held in the early evening when clients were most likely to be about.

The 'studio' was the shelter's dining room, situated next to the 'wet' TV room (where alcohol could be consumed) with access to a side-room with a sink. This location created considerable footfall. When no clients were in the session, I would sit using the materials as this often attracted the interest of passers-by who would ask me what I was doing. I had researched into how the art therapist can be a participant observer for my MA thesis and would, depending on circumstances, continue with mark making during the session (Richardson, 1997). As people were continually being moved on attendance could be for just a single session, normally it was three or four; where someone needed more specific accommodation it could be up to ten.

One session

Barry worked throughout on a painting based on a photograph of the Cornish coastline in a book he had brought. He seemed absorbed in this even though other people around him were talking. Anja kept saying she was concerned because her boyfriend had not been at the hospital when she went to visit him that morning. She had no idea where he might be. Barry suggested she report him to the police as missing. Ricky worked on a card for his new girlfriend. He asked me to draw the outline of a flower, which he carefully coloured in and decorated. Mike sat with a can of lager and a piece of paper. Intermittently he would do some drawing, then talk to Ricky or me about what he had done. The drawings were of different 'characters' and he speculated about who they might be and what they were doing. He was frustrated at how shaky his hand was. Anja did some fashion designs but found it difficult to concentrate because of her worries about her boyfriend. An ambulance crew arrived for Mike and asked him to return to hospital with them. He had discharged himself earlier in the day after having hit his head on the pavement when he had a fall. As the session ended Barry asked if he could continue working on his painting. I explained he could sign out the art materials from the office whenever he wanted to use them. After the session staff on shift told me that Anja's boyfriend had died the day before. She had been removed by hospital security that morning having become distressed because he was not there.

Studio art therapy offered a creative and social meeting place for people who otherwise had no access to art-based or other activities. Interaction with the space could be tentative as many were living with enduring mental health issues, trauma, or the physical or neurological effects of substance use. Yet every week people still came along, as the sessions offered a place where they were met as individuals rather than 'clients with support needs'. With attendance sometimes for just a single session, interaction was very much in the here and now. Studio art therapy set a context for a nexus of relations around both the creative process and what was made. Work could be seen to index someone's current situation, such as Mike's drawings being shaky through alcohol use and concussion, or how they used the space to exercise individual and creative agency, such as Barry's paintings. Over time, as people passed through the sessions, this required holding in mind many different life stories and experiences.

An accommodation-based project

Comprising part of a 'recovery pathway' for people with mental health and substance-use issues, the project provided accommodation to twenty-one residents for a period of up to two years. Aside from the laundry there were no communal rooms and residents seldom interacted with each other. Art therapy was scheduled as one of a number of onsite activities, offering people an alternative to watching TV alone in their rooms or going out to buy alcohol or drugs. Sessions were held in the early evening when clients were most likely to be about.

The 'studio' was a newly built activities room in the project's garden which could comfortably accommodate up to eight people, had a sink, cupboards for storing materials, and space to display work. I would sit using the materials until people arrived, putting them aside to signal they had my attention. Attendance at the sessions was more consistent as people could be resident in the project for up to two years. Clients had a local borough connection and reflected its diverse multicultural population.

One session

Luke looked in first and, having made clear he was not staying, sat drinking a can of ginger beer while explaining the finer points of begging. Following his departure others began to arrive. Teddy picked one or two objects for me to arrange and then drew them with coloured crayons. Always certain anything he did would be 'useless' he was pleasantly surprised at the outcome. I held up his drawing so he could view it from a distance. He judged it good enough to be added to the display on the wall. Filipe used water-soluble pencils to draw a picture of the Indian island where he grew up, remembering picking fruit off trees and catching fish in the ocean. He talked about coming to the UK in the 1980s, hoping to find a better life but instead being dogged by addiction and depression. He yearned to return to his birthplace but no longer had any family there. Marcia made a card for her youngest son (who was living with his father's family) colouring in the message 'Welcome Home'. She asked me to keep count while she went through the names of her children. She felt sure there were six but could only remember five. She loved thinking about them coming to visit her once she was 'clean' and settled in a flat. Irshad drew series' of images and this time he did a tree drawing. The tree's trunk always had a large gash in it, which looked like some kind of wound. He explained that he liked watching nature programmes on TV and loved the way birds made nests in holes they found in trees. He wanted to find somewhere secure like that.

Studio art therapy in the project evolved its own sense of community. The content of work was rarely spoken about directly (even if I asked about some aspect of it) but still generated conversation. People would talk about issues they were facing, and others would share their own similar experiences. How the work functioned depended on how someone felt able to be with it. Irshad's relationship to his work could be about it as an object (the composition, colours, and shapes), an activity to take his mind off his anxiety, a place of fantasy or escape and, sometimes, allowing it to echo experiences from his adolescence (he had come to the UK as a refugee). Marcia's cards for her son were created with great care but also enabled her to have some tangible sense of connection to him in his absence. Through being seen as an index of the person and their experience, work (and the person) could be engaged with at multiple and differing levels.

Recovery college

Set up in 2012, the recovery college had a focus on co-production and client-led or co-facilitated activities. I ran studio art therapy sessions from its inception, but the 'Creative Art and Art Therapy' I describe here ran from April 2016 to November 2018. It was co-produced with a volunteer with lived experience of homelessness; she ran workshops on creative art activities like marbling or print-making while I facilitated a space where people could do work of their own. Each term we agreed a programme of workshops she would run, meeting after every session for an informal debrief.

The 'studio' was a large multi-use training room that could accommodate up to forty people, with plenty of storage space and a kitchenette. The size of the room meant there could be an area for creative art activities and another for art therapy. People moved between each area depending on how they wanted to use the session, with many working in the liminal space in between. I refrained from participating in art making so as to circulate and be available for people as needed. A core group of five or six people attended regularly (with a sessional average of twelve) with sessions running for three hours on Thursday afternoons.

One session

Pete unpacked pencils and a sketchbook from his bag. He had found a picture in a newspaper that he wanted to draw and set to work. Later on I sat with him, and we looked through his sketchbook together. He recalled when and where each draw-ing had been done, picking out the ones he felt had worked best. Stewart asked me to photocopy an outline drawing of a pheasant, which he carefully coloured in with water-soluble pencils. He then used them to do a free-hand drawing of the recovery college adding in all the people he liked meeting there. After this he made a coffee and sat watching the others working till the session ended. Niamh had asked the previous week for some acrylic medium to be bought. Mixing it with paints she began applying fluid, saturated colours to a sheet of A2 watercol-our paper. As she worked she talked about the composition and how it was devel-oping, seeing religious associations in one of the figure-like shapes. Grace spent some time looking through magazines for ideas, but nothing appealed. Eventu-ally she decided just to start applying acrylic paint to an A3 canvas and from these tentative marks a woman's face began to emerge. When it was finished she sat contemplating the work and, once it was dry, carefully wrapped it up to take home with her. Akram came over when the printmaking workshop ended. Apply-ing acrylic paint to his polystyrene 'block' of a bird in flight he made several prints, painting into each one by hand and letting different ideas evolve. He liked the spontaneity of this process and shared with me some of the associations these images generated for him.

Creative art and art therapy in combination showed how art and art making, even in a learning-based context, can never be just about gaining skills. However directive a workshop may be 'learners' still feel invested in their work; in Gell's terms it is part of their distributed personhood. How their work is responded to is therefore crucial. What art therapy gave to these sessions was an openness to peoples' emotional ambivalence to and about their work (and by extension them-selves). Pete's sketchbook or Grace's paintings were not simply evidence of skills or potentially symbolic (though they could be both) but distributed aspects of themselves. The continual interplay between 'creative art' and 'art therapy', like Akram's printmaking, challenged assumptions about what either might be and when they might be happening. Nonpictorial or abstract work could be approached as potentially meaningful through being relatively replete and indexing that person's creativity. For people attending the sessions (and by extension their work), this provided an environment in which creativity and personal experience could coalesce and be explored.

Exhibition: seeing and being seen

I have focused so far on studio art therapy as an environment in which work can be made, but it is equally somewhere that work can be seen. Work made in sessions was not only visible during its making but could potentially be displayed in the studio or other places. Case and Dalley characterise the process of looking at images in art therapy as 'responding aesthetically' to the work made (2014: 106). This 'aesthetic experience', mediated and informed by psychoanalytic theories of art, facilitates an understanding of the image's symbolic content and meaning (2014: 250). Yet one aspect of 'art' being a contested term is that how it is looked at (or interacted with) similarly becomes contingent. I therefore want to revisit the process of looking at work in art therapy, particularly what can happen when it is displayed or exhibited.

Being seen

While terms like 'display' or 'exhibition' invite associations with galleries and questions of value, it is the social relations they can facilitate with and around art that I want to focus on. This has a particular resonance in the context of homelessness where people have often sat alone on a street unnoticed by passers-by. Exhibition can then incorporate a quality of being seen for both the work and the person who made it. Joe attended art therapy at the rolling shelter. Having grown up in care, he had lived on and off the streets for twenty years. He liked working on grey pastel paper because it was like the paving stones he drew on when he was street homeless. Making art on the pavement made him some money and created a way into conversation with passers-by. He told me how talking with people about his work helped break his isolation; they in turn saw him in a completely different way.

The rolling shelter had nowhere to display work done in studio art therapy, reflecting the transience of the setting. In one session, Steve did a small drawing he called 'Rudy I miss U'. It was an outline of a dog's head with the message underneath. Steve's dog Rudy had been stolen and every attempt to find him had failed. Steve talked about how bereft he felt and as he left the session he fixed his drawing to the wall. In that anonymous space it barely noticed, but it was a poignant trace of Rudy and the bond they had shared. The drawing remained there, untouched, until Steve collected it when he moved out. It's staying in place when other things were torn down suggested how much it had resonated with others. The work indexed Rudy's being taken, but in displaying it Steve had marked not just his particular loss but the ubiquity of loss in the lives of homeless people.

Looking back

The studio at the homeless project did have a display space, with a changing body of work on show. Yet this was not simply a rolling exhibition but constituted a distributed object, individually and collectively, of the people who came to the sessions. They were able to see their work and by extension themselves from a different viewpoint. When Filipe completed a drawing we would look at it together and, if he wanted it to be added to the display, discuss where it might best fit. I would hold it next to other pieces of his work for him to see. As this happened aspects of the new piece might echo or amplify parts of earlier works; connections could be explored. Viewing his work in this way offered him many levels of engaging with it and by extension aspects of himself.

Collectively, the work on display reflected the vitality of the sessions, the work made, and the time spent together. As it evolved and grew, this body of work became a resource as well as a record. While art books and other visual material were available to use, the display seemed more resonant through its indexing the creativity and experiences of people living through similar situations. Even after someone had moved on, their presence was still evidenced through the work they had made. In a setting where people often lack access to resources this display could simultaneously evidence and motivate their agency.

Being shown

In the recovery college, people could have their work framed and displayed in the studio, around the building, or sometimes in external exhibition spaces. Beyond simply showing their work, this involved them in a particular kind of social relations with others. Gell describes encountering an art object as coming into contact with the distributed mind and agency of the person who made it. As Sansi explains, this references anthropological theories of 'the gift' in which, through gifts, people give (aspects of) themselves to others (2015: 97). This counters the aesthetic paradigm of art as a passive object of contemplation (which informs the standardised model) the limitations of which Carroll (1999) and Sansi (2015) elucidate. Peoples' work could engage viewers not just as captivating objects but also, as Steve's drawing of Rudy had done, as ways to share and mark experience.

Display or exhibition in this context involved a quality of how someone (through their work) was seen and how others were, literally, affected by having seen it. Mitchell characterises images not as 'passive entities' but as living things that 'change the way we think and see and dream' (2005: 92). Goodman identifies them as 'ways of worldmaking' through which people can explore and communicate experience (1978: 106). People attending 'Creative Art and Art Therapy' could (and did) show work in the recovery college's open access client-led arts magazine; in cafés around London with a community arts group; and with major London galleries like the Royal Academy of Arts, which offer outreach sessions to homelessness charities (and provided workshops in Creative Art and Art Therapy). Exhibiting in these settings enabled people, their work, and life experiences to be seen and acknowledged.

When is art therapy?

A theme of this chapter has been that the standardised model of the image fits awkwardly with studio art therapy. It involves art making, but its structure is linguistic through being informed by theory and practice from a range of linguistically based psychological therapies. The relationship between image and word is framed, as Mitchell describes it, in 'extracting the hidden verbal message from the inarticulate pictorial surface' (1987: 45). There is a way in which the historical tension between word and image he discusses is played out in art therapy, with the image in word-centred practice prioritised over the image in art-centred practice. Art or art making outside the standardised model is often described as being 'healing' or calming, something which can equally be claimed for any number of activities.

The studio art therapy sessions in homelessness services involved an openness to the different ways 'art' can be meaningful. Attending to work as relatively replete and indexical of each person made engagement possible through every aspect of it. This was particularly valuable in these services where many people were living with complex mental and physical health issues, their first language might not be English, and they were not necessarily familiar with the concept of art being 'about' something. Recognising 'art' as extending beyond what the standardised model allows for enabled me to be open to the therapeutic potential in the interactions and communication that 'art' and its making facilitated. I was able to engage with clients through this multiplicity of creativity by focusing on 'when' (rather than 'what') is art therapy. Studio art therapy provided a framework that could accommodate this approach, opening up new possibilities for art therapy practice in the process.

References

Carroll, N. (1999) *Philosophy of Art, a Contemporary Introduction.* Abingdon: Routledge.
Case, C. and Dalley, T. (2014) *The Handbook of Art Therapy,* Third edition. London: Routledge.
Gaiger, J. (2008) *Aesthetics and Painting.* London: Continuum International Publishing Group.
Gell, A. (1998) *Art and Agency, An Anthropological Theory.* Oxford: Oxford University Press.
Goodman, N. (1976) *Languages of Art: An Approach to the Theory of Symbols,* Second Edition. Indianapolis: Hackett.
Goodman, N. (1978) *Ways of Worldmaking.* Indianapolis: Hackett.

Hatt, M. and Klonk, C. (2006) *Art History: A Critical Introduction to its Methods*. Manchester: Manchester University Press.

Mitchell, W. (1986) *Iconology: Image, Text, Ideology*. Chicago: The University of Chicago Press.

Mitchell, W. (2005) *What Do Pictures Want? The Lives and Loves of Images*. Chicago: The University of Chicago Press.

Moon, C.H. (2002) *Studio Art Therapy: Cultivating the Artist Identity in the Art Therapist*. London and Philadelphia: Jessica Kingsley Publishers.

Richardson, S. (1997) *Colourful Language: Examining the Role of Participant Observer in Art Therapy*. MA Dissertation, University of Hertfordshire.

Richardson, S. (2015) Completing the picture: Art therapy with a client with ME. In Liebmann, M. and Weston, S. (eds.) *Art Therapy with Physical Conditions*. London: Jessica Kingsley Publishers.

Sansi, R. (2015) *Art, Anthropology and The Gift*. London: Bloomsbury.

Warburton, N. (2003) *The Art Question*. London: Routledge.

19 Reliquary for the departed

Archiving and collections

Christopher Brown and Helen Omand

The etymological roots of 'reliquary' contain 'remaining' and 'leave behind' as pertaining to objects of interest due to age or association. In art therapy the material object is the artwork, which may be left behind for various reasons. Art therapy departments in the old psychiatric hospitals during the period 1945–2000 accumulated large volumes of patients' artwork that had been left behind. Inevitably, a time would come when these had to be disposed of due to closure of the institution or the department. What to do with these accumulations of images? Edward Adamson, a pioneer art therapist who worked at Netherne Hospital between 1945 and 1981, allegedly amassed 100,000 pictures, which on his departure he whittled down to a personal collection of over 5,000 (Timlin, 2014) and shortly afterwards, the hospital authorities disposed of the remainder in skips (O'Flynn et al., 2018). In 2015, the majority of work from his collection was given over to the care of the Wellcome Collection.

Of course, the problem may be solved by not accumulating images in the first place – a position currently endorsed by the British Association of Art Therapists (2021). Changing attitudes to keeping artworks have arisen through a lack of storage space in modern settings and different ethics of ownership and privacy. Historical associations with psychiatric collections and outsider art contain the uneasy power dynamics of Western medical and art history practices, where the marginalised may be profited from. It is no wonder the profession of art therapy has sought to distance itself from this history.

In this chapter, we consider what value might be placed on the relics left behind in art therapy once the client has departed and, perhaps controversially, what potential value there may still be in collecting, archiving, and exhibiting them. We take as a case example the conundrum of a portfolio of artwork collected by art therapist Myra Cohen from her work with patients in the 1970s at Hill End Hospital. Thinking about historical collections in relation to current practices opens up questions around future cultural knowledge and how this may be transmitted.

DOI: 10.4324/9781003095606-23

Collecting

Take a walk along a beach, your eyes scan the sand and spot a piece of sea glass or a pleasingly patterned shell, you pick it up and place it in your pocket. As you continue walking, this is added to by other pieces that catch your eye. Emptying your pocket on returning home you place these objects on a shelf – you have a collection.

Theories about collecting are to be found in the disciplines of psychology and cultural studies. We do not intend to explore these in any depth, merely to give a taste of the subject before turning to collections of artworks from psychiatric settings.

Freud, in his short paper titled 'Character and Anal Eroticism' (1908) links collecting to parsimony and the desire to retain. Gamwell (1996), writing about Freud's own collection of antiquities, likens his collecting and his irresistible impulse to acquire new pieces to his addiction to cigar smoking.

Jean Baudrillard, a cultural theorist within postmodernity, says: 'It should be stressed that the concept of collecting (from the Latin *colligere*, to select and assemble) is distinct from that of accumulating' (1994: 22). He points out the active phase of collecting by children between the ages of seven and twelve and suggests a correlation with sexuality through a compensatory function. He goes on to emphasise the seriality of the acquisition of objects and links this to desire and possession that is ultimately a discourse oriented towards oneself.

Susan Pearce, in her seminal analysis of the subject 'Museums, Objects and Collections' neatly combines both approaches when she says:

> The process of selection lies at the heart of collecting, and as we shall see, the act of collecting is not simple; it involves both a view of inherited social ideas of the value which should (or should not) be attached to a particular object and which derive from the modern narratives we have been considering, and impulses which lie at the deepest level of individual personality.
>
> (1992: 7)

David Maclagan, writing about outsider art (2009), suggests there was a 'classic' period of psychotic art:

> Historically bracketed between the closing decades of the nineteenth century, when the first collections of patient art were established and books began to be published trying to make sense of it in other than purely diagnostic terms, and the period after the second world war when changes in psychiatric treatment, such as shorter hospital stays, the use of more sophisticated anti-psychotic medication and the provision of art therapy, diluted conditions that made it possible for such work to meet the criteria for authentic Art Brut.
>
> (2009: 75)

The importance of authenticity was to feed the emerging art world market for such pieces following the establishment of the genre of Art Brut by the artist Jean Dubuffet. Psychotic art formed over half his initial collection, taken as 'abandoned goods' from psychiatric hospitals in the aftermath of the Second World War (Maclagan, 2009). Artist collections like that of Dubuffet, with its focus on authentic artistic creativity and links to the art market, are in contrast to the medical collections of psychiatrists such as Prinzhorn in the 1920s, where the focus is human curiosity. Collecting, where it stands outside of an economic system such as the global art market, is intrinsically bound up with curiosity and classification.

However, both artistic and medical collections might involve power dynamics of the 'sophisticated' viewer/knowledge holder marvelling at something uncivilised, primitive, and 'other'. In Art Brut there is an idea of something untainted – a 'pure' artistic expression being revered, which is sometimes rather like the medical or archaeological collector displaying a cabinet of curiosities to a peer group or appreciative society. In both cases the original artist may be unaware of the value of their work as it is transported from one world into another. The relationship of 'collector' to 'collected' is power infused, as the collector decides what has value – either to themselves or a like-minded audience. When the things collected are not shells or pebbles, but cultural products made by human hands, problems of pathology and exploitation may be present. Prinz (2017) suggests further ethical problems; for the collection to retain value, the marginalised must be kept marginalised and societal binaries of inside/outside are reinforced. As a profession, perhaps we are a bit ashamed of any associations with Art Brut now and fall over ourselves to show that we aren't curious voyeurs, we are not making aesthetic judgements, collecting for our own pleasure or for the favour of our audiences.

Curating

Maclagan suggests that there was 'a gradual process of cultural erosion' (2009: 108) as ideas about confidentiality from art therapy practice took hold in psychiatric institutions. A 'sealing in' (Ibid.) of the artwork produced in such places, away from the public eye and economic exploitation. Thus, a new and dominant culture emerged as art therapy became increasingly aligned with psychotherapy, which privileged the sanctity of the therapeutic relationship. Adamson had no such qualms about exhibiting works from his collection in a purpose-built gallery within the hospital, although only open to selected visitors (Adamson, 1984). On his retirement, this gallery was dismantled by the institution and the collection had to be rescued by friends who set up a charitable trust, one of whom, Dr Miriam Rothschild opened a public gallery on her estate near Cambridge for its display (Timlin, 1983).

That the institution had no interest in looking after Adamson's collection seems surprising. Perhaps there were some ethical concerns by a medical establishment used to patient confidentiality, or perhaps they simply didn't care. Curating has its

Latin root in *curare*, to take care of. In Roman times it was a role of civic care-taker, in the medieval period that of a priest taking care of the souls of a parish, and in the late eighteenth century that of looking after a museum collection. Its contemporary meaning has expanded to include preservation, selection, research, and making exhibitions (Obrist, 2014).

What happened to all the other accumulated 'collections' in the old psychiatric hospitals dotted around the country? David Edwards has written about his experience of dealing with such an accumulation when he left his post as art therapist in Stanley Royd Hospital. What to do with the hundreds of images was not only problematical in terms of which to save and which to discard but also because of the emotion evoked by the task: '*These images, these pictures, what are they to me now? I don't know. The subject of a future article, lecture, the germ of an idea, a memory, transitional objects (something to hold onto), something dead returned to haunt me?*' (1997: 53 italics in original). Edwards wonders about his current relationship to these 'relics' of the therapeutic relationship in a way that evokes traces of past events. This potential for images to reanimate the past depends on an appreciation of the context in which they were made. But this sets up a tension between the historical and aesthetic aspects of the artwork (Brown et al., 2017). Exhibitions of images made in therapeutic settings often present their aesthetic value as outside the context of its production and thus the audience is expected to view them as art on a par with any other art object. Is there something disingenuous about such an approach? The power of such images may be due to raw emotion finding form – not so sublimated as that of the conventional artist. Their power may be as much to disturb as to delight.

Archiving

How do we assess the value of an archive of works from art therapy? Anthropologists and ethnographers have used the term 'affordance' to describe the possibilities held by a work or collection – what it allows a person to do/think/react in interaction with it. 'Affordances are the ways in which things come into the immediate presence of perceivers, not as objects-in-themselves, closed in and contained, but in their potential for the continuation of a form of life' (Ingold, 2018: 39). In this view, the artwork is not a static object but holds latent potential for future interactions. We use a vignette from our own experience by way of example.

Vignette

Chris sets the scene.

A large, black canvas portfolio sits on the table in my studio. It contains a collection of 35mm slides, original artworks, and ephemera that belonged to an artist, Myra Cohen, who worked in the art therapy department at Hill End

Hospital, Hertfordshire from 1968 to 1986. Before she died, Myra gave the collection to Philippa Brown who was then course leader for the MA Art Therapy at the University of Hertfordshire. Her wish was for it to have a custodian who would understand and respect the images it contained. With the collection came both a responsibility and a dilemma, how to care for it and what to do with it. As I had become interested in the question of collections and archives through the Adamson collection, I offered to take a closer look at it. And now here it is, sitting on my table, patiently waiting for me to open it. Of course, this is not quite the opening of Tutankhamen's tomb, but I am aware of the need to systematically catalogue what I shall find inside. I have entered the world of archiving, a land inhabited by people obsessed by detail and classification. I feel at home.

Helen brings a slide projector.

We are curious to discover what the affordance of this collection might be for us, fifty years on from its original conception. We use an old analogue carousel projector to view the 86 slides that are the core of the collection along with Cohen's handwritten notes about each. They are organised as series from six patients, the first of which comprises nearly half the slides. The carousel whirrs into life and the images spring into focus in the darkness. The qualities of projected light hold a somewhat ephemeral feeling; a moment in time brought into the present on our screen. As we view the images one by one, starting with a psychedelic abstract of swirling lines (Figure 19.1), we were initially uncertain about what to say. Our first spontaneous comments in response were, perhaps inevitably, speculative about any potential symbolism or meaning and it is remarkable how strong this pull to interpret, to be 'a therapist' can be. Cohen's notes were minimal with just a very brief history of admission. Mostly, she recorded what the patient said about each picture with occasional comments on the aesthetic qualities by herself.

We eventually moved to a position of reflecting on our reactions as audience. After a seemingly endless succession of images by the same patient we confessed to feeling unmoved by his pictures, which conveyed distress in graphic terms but with little compelling aesthetic (Figure 19.2). We linked this to the absence of a personal story with which to contextualise it. We felt a sense of guilt that immense loss and human suffering must be present, but it was hard to feel it. This led to a rather voyeuristic quality to our viewing, disconnected from any emotional impact and compounded by the control afforded by the forward button on the projector. The active decision to press it and move on, 'next!' felt more pronounced than in an exhibition where one might naturally wander past some pictures and stop at others. We then had a realisation that this patient's particular state of mind was of course affecting us through his work, leaving us 'flat'. Its power to do so raises questions about the presence of the original maker in an artwork.

Viewing further sets of images, which seemed to be arranged chronologically from beginning to end of therapy, brought an awareness that Myra's original

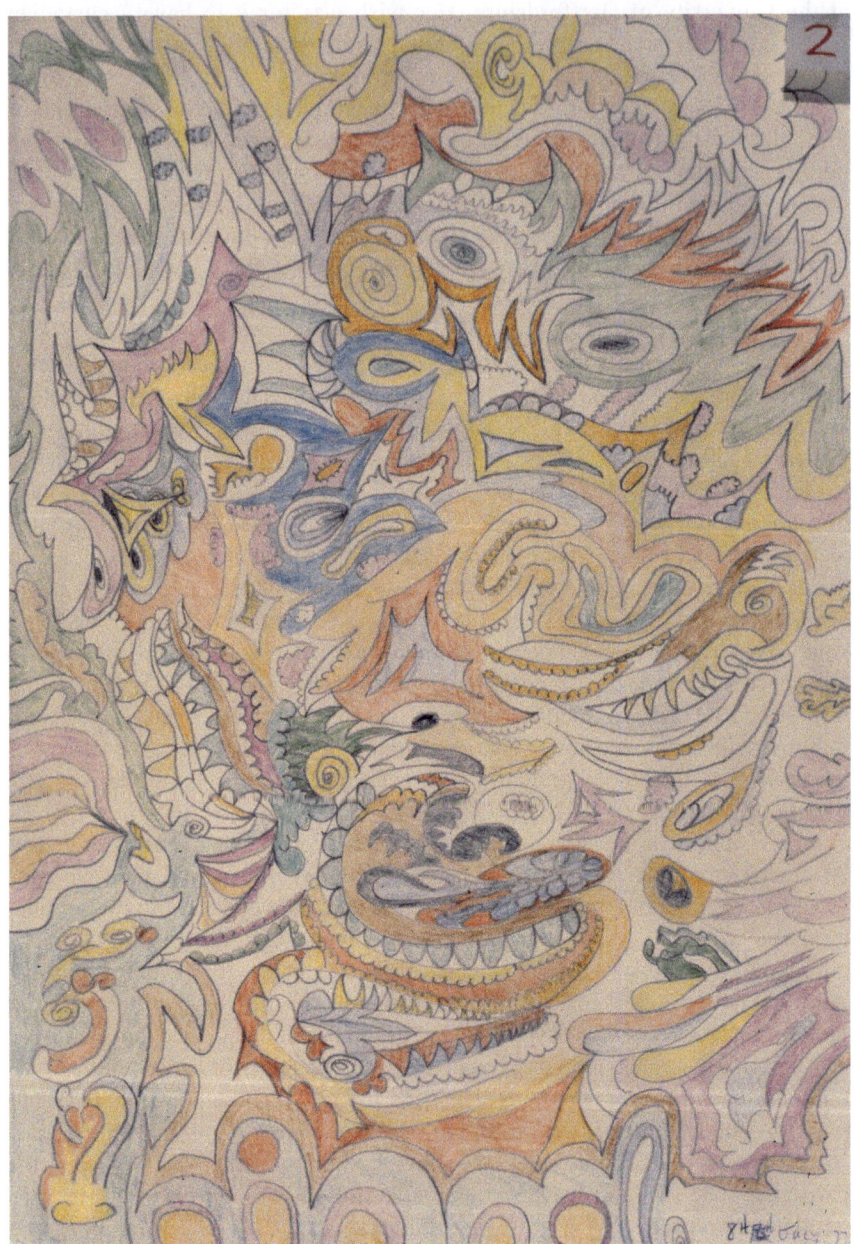

Figure 19.1 Original creator unknown.

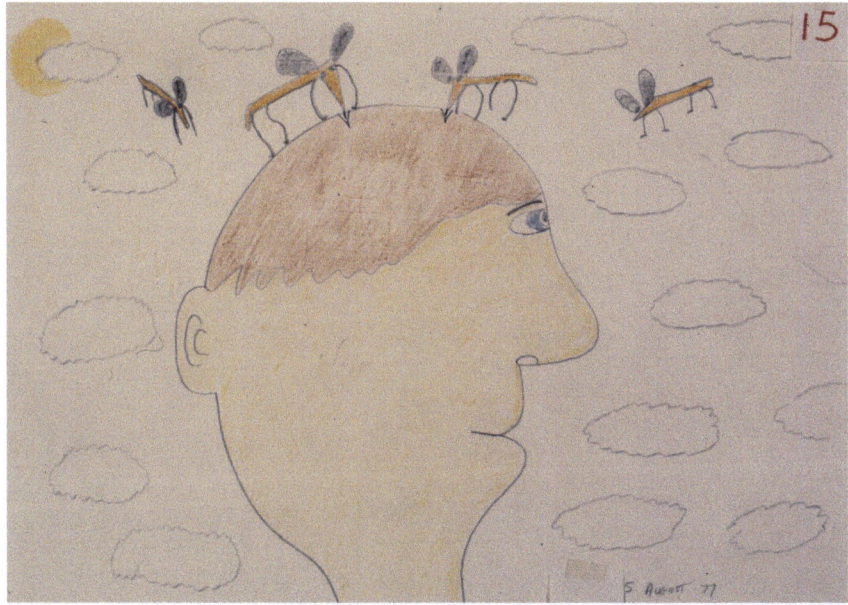

Figure 19.2 Original creator unknown.

purpose for these was undoubtedly to convey, to the medical establishment, proof of improvement and the part played by art therapy in patients' recovery. Historically, this tells us about art therapy's positioning in the psychiatry department. Finally, in complete contrast, the last two sets presented us unexpectedly with images that, in their power to communicate something of the artist's distress, were startling and moving. We felt these could stand on their own as art, without any backstory, due to their visual impact (Figures 19.3 & 19.4).

We felt that we had experienced artwork from two ends of a spectrum – those whose meaning resided more in the therapeutic relationship and those whose meaning could exist outside of that relationship due to their artistic aesthetic. In contrast to the rich visual nature of the latter, the set of diagram-like images of the former conveyed something of the painful monotony of mental illness, away from the glamourised 'psychotic art' with its countercultural associations. This led us to think about the value of both contrasting portraits of people undergoing mental distress and perhaps our own bias towards the thrill of art that communicates vividly. We can only guess how Myra Cohen felt about them in the context of their relationship, but seeing them out of their context made us wonder what is it that is intriguing or distasteful for the individual viewer, and what does it tell us about our culturally wired predispositions towards certain accepted aesthetics.

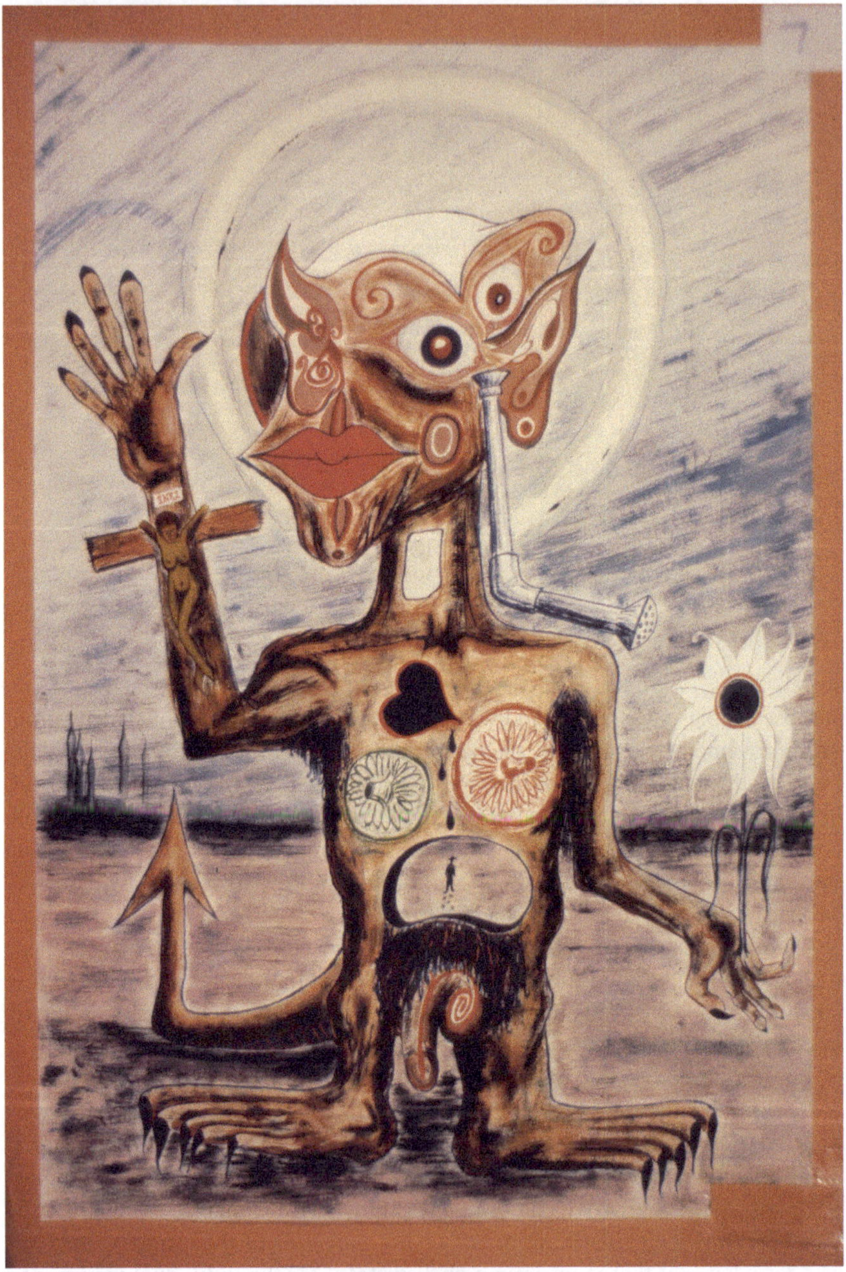

Figure 19.3 Original creator unknown.

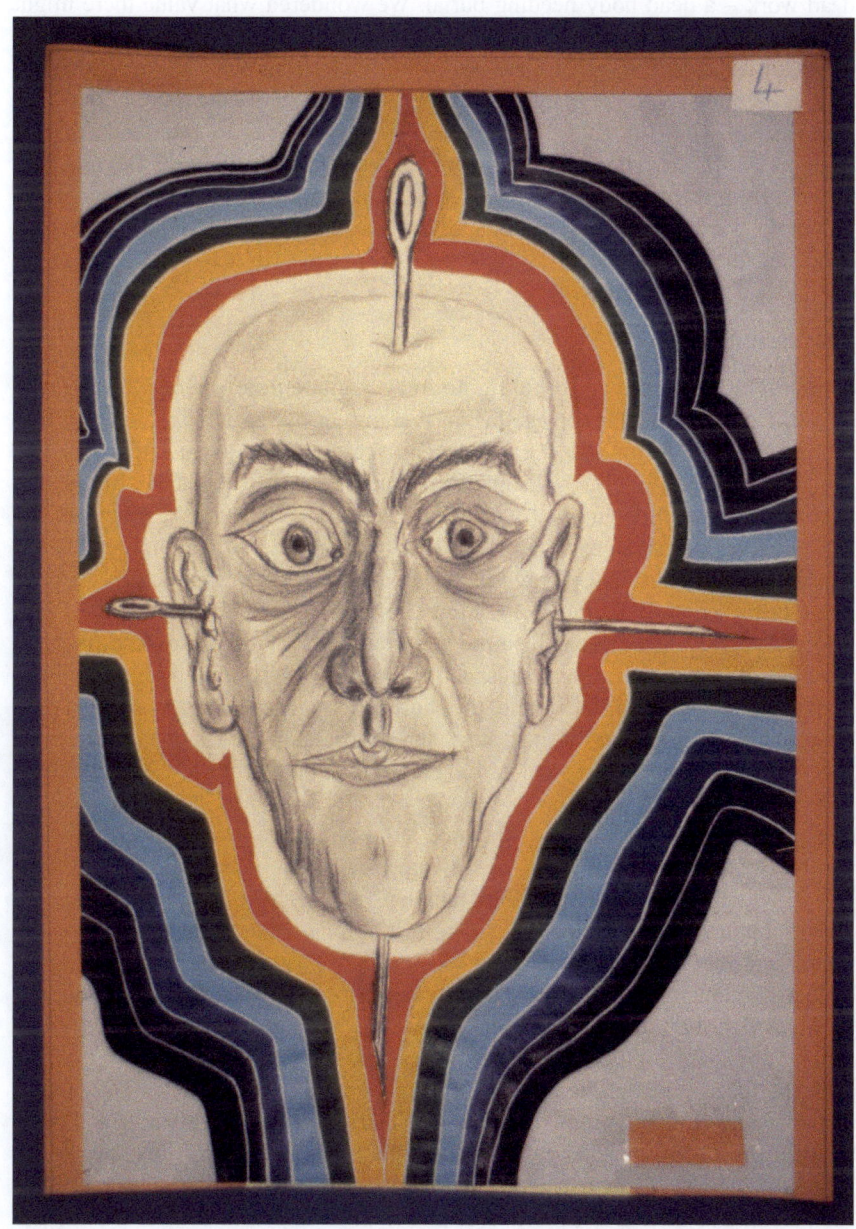

Figure 19.4 Original creator unknown.

Our viewing raised questions about why we keep work made in art therapy. In a sense, the work, outside of the relational context in which it was made, is dead work – a dead body needing burial. We wondered what value there might be in such a collection as a 'cultural product'. The affordance of the viewing for us, as art therapists, was that it enabled us to think, from a professional perspective, about how we value images and the problems with taking them out of their context. But what value might the collection have if seen by the public on, for example, a website showcasing a historical aspect of art therapy? Beyond permission from the patient what ethical issues arise from the context and nature of the viewing experience? We examine these questions in the next section, which concludes the chapter.

Discussion

Why might we be drawn to hold onto images made in art therapy? The art is a record of the work done together in therapy. Is there, perhaps, a sense that the pictures half-belong to the setting and the therapist, as an intersubjective product? (Skaife, 2008). A therapist may not want to throw out objects that have been powerfully imbued with meaning. Schaverien (1987) describes the scapegoat and talisman as two possibilities of meaning that may influence their safekeeping and disposal. There may be an appreciation of the picture's former value to the client in therapy, or it might be kept out of a regard for the client. Coming across old work can be a poignant reminder of the person and the relationship. It can seem rather disrespectful to throw away something *of* another person, once so valued. Of course, the short-term nature of therapy in most psychiatric hospitals now, with short stays and short session times, may mean there is less time for clients to spend making art or for the therapist to get 'attached' to them or to the art.

The 'accumulating' phase seems to be more of a 'care taking' function where the image is carefully put away for 'safe keeping' in its natural home in the context in which it was made and thus functions as part of a holding environment (Winnicott, 1965). The selecting and collecting phase seems more active as the image is moved into a different context. The act of changing the context and purpose of the images, with the potential for separation between aesthetics and personal history, may set up uneasy tensions as it is here that power dynamics come into it – the image will be 'used' for a new purpose.

In the aforementioned example, the purpose of the images Myra Cohen collected appears to have been educational, primarily for the psychiatrists and other medical personnel, in order to show the efficacy of art therapy. Our own experience of viewing them had elements of the following: feeling distanced from the person and their story, a sense of power in having control over the images (via the projector), indulging in speculation around meaning and diagnosis. These seemed to echo something of what we know of the dynamic aspects of the method employed by the psychiatrists Cunningham Dax and Reitman at Netherne, who were brought images from the art therapy studio run by Edward Adamson, for them to draw conclusions about their creators' mental illness (Reitman, 1950; Cunningham Dax, 1953). We need to be careful therefore about the potential for pathologising that may come with a tendency to link what we know of a person's diagnosis, with the content and form of their images, without them being present to tell us what they meant.

The audience also needs consideration. What is it about art from outside of the mainstream that people wish to see? For example, is the audience who visit the annual Koestler Exhibition (koestlerarts.org.uk) of artwork from prisons thrilled by a glimpse of an 'other' world on the edges of society, usually hidden from view? Perhaps the artwork holds the unwanted 'mad', 'bad' parts of ourselves and, by locating it there, our comfortable status as insiders may be reaffirmed. Or are we looking for something else, perhaps an affirmation of the disturbance in all of us? We go to be moved in some way. Is this in a different way to conventional art exhibitions or similar? Here context is everything:

> There are also many disturbing and difficult to look at images in the contemporary art world, for example Tracy Emin's 'My Bed' (1998) or Jake and Dinos Chapman's 'Hell' (1998–2000). The Chapman brother's 'Hell' might be seen very differently if it was viewed in a social context that emphasized a lack of integration and rationality, i.e. madness, as opposed to one of an avant-garde in art.
>
> (Brown, 2017: 4)

The artworks in art therapy may be taken care of, over time, by the therapist and thus be part of a curating function. They may be kept by the therapist as a collection, which may be used for educational purpose such as a case study, a lecture, or for public exhibition in a gallery. These activities will be mostly of a contemporary nature with permission given by the patient. But what happens when such collections become historical artefacts? Should they be archived and therefore available for future generations of art therapists to look at and think about? If so, whose hands would they be in and who has the power to decide how they are seen? How might service users be involved? Returning to the idea of affordances, contexts such as museums and exhibitions activate historical collections, which can then become catalysts for intercultural understanding, recovering lost narratives, and raising ethical issues with new audiences.

At the beginning of this chapter we referred to the Edward Adamson Collection at the Wellcome Collection. We wondered how this resource was being used. There was a public consultation about the collection in 2017 with an event titled 'Art, Power and the Asylum: Exploring the Adamson Collection' (see O'Flynn et al., 2018), which addressed ethical questions arising from the way value, power, and identity shape how the collection is framed. Issues of ownership and copyright are problematic when hospital records have been destroyed and the Wellcome see themselves as 'guardians' of the work (2018: 397). Regarding naming of the original creator, the dilemma hinges on whether 'anonymity can be construed as dehumanising' (p 398), and O'Flynn states that the discussion 'made it clear that there are no easy answers when it comes to publishing the names of those we know little or nothing about' (p 399). A recurring question was about whether these works should be seen as art or medical records, along with their opposing contexts of exhibition or confidentiality. Although O'Flynn states 'objects such as those Adamson collected can be, simultaneously, artefacts of mental health and art therapy history, documents of therapeutic experiences, and works of art' (p 396), the idea that art therapy might claim more than a historical footnote in this debate is absent. We suggest that this debate is not only embedded in the history of the profession of art therapy but also needs to be brought more fully into the discourse of contemporary practice.

References

Adamson, E. (1984) *Art as Healing*. Coventure, London.

BAAT. (2021) Advice on storing and keeping artworks and clinical notes after the end of therapy. Available at: www.baat.org/Membership/Documents/Professional-Advice. Accessed 01.09.2020.

Baudrillard, J. (1994) The system of collecting. In: *The cultures of collecting*, Elsner, J. and Cardinal, R. (Eds.). Reaktion Books, London.

Brown, C. (2017) Inside out: Thoughts about the frame in art therapy. *ATOL: Art Therapy OnLine*, 8 (1). Available at: https://journals.gold.ac.uk/index.php/atol/article/view/444/pdf.

Brown, C., Martyn, J. and Skaife, S. (2017) Exhibition review. *ATOL: Art Therapy OnLine*, 8 (2). Available at: https://journals.gold.ac.uk/index.php/atol/article/view/464/pdf.

Dax, E. Cunningham. (1953) *Experimental studies in psychiatric art*. Faber, London.

Edwards, D. (1997) Endings. *Inscape: The Journal of the British Association of Art Therapists*, 2 (2): 49–56.

Freud, S. (1908) Character and anal eroticism. *Standard Edition* (1959), 9: 167–175.

Gamwell, L. (1996) A collector analyses collecting: Sigmund Freud on the passion to possess. In: *Excavations and their objects: Freud's collection of antiquity*, Barker, S. (Ed.). State University of New York Press, Albany.

Ingold, T. (2018) Back to the future with the theory of affordances. *FHAU: Journal of Ethnographic Theory*, 8 (1/2): 39–44.

Koestler Arts www.koestlerarts.org.uk/exhibitions/.

Maclagan, D. (2009) *Outsider art. From the margins to the marketplace*. Reaktion Books, London.

Obrist, H. U. (2015) *Ways of curating*. Penguin Edition, London.

O'Flynn, D., Szekir – Papasavva, S. and Trainor, C. (2018) Art, power, and the asylum: Adamson, healing, and the collection. *The Lancet*, 5 (5): 396–369.

Pearce, S. M. (1992) *Museums, objects and collections: A cultural study*. Leicester University Press, London.

Prinz, J. (2017) Against outsider art. *Journal of Social Philosophy*, 48 (3): 250–273.

Reitman, F. (1950). *Psychotic art*. Routledge, London.

Schaverien, J. (1987) The scapegoat and the talisman: Transference in art therapy. In: *Images of art therapy new developments in theory and practice*, Dalley, T. et al. (Eds.). Routledge, London.

Skaife, S. (2008) Off-shore: A deconstruction of David Maclagan's and David Mann's 'inscape' papers. *International Journal of Art Therapy: Inscape*, 13 (2).

Timlin, J. (1983) An apple for the teacher. In: *Art as healing* (1984). Adamson, E. Coventure, London.

Timlin, J. (2014) *Preface to 2014 reissue of art as healing.* Wellcome Library, London.

Winnicott, D. W. (1965) *The maturational processes and the facilitating environment.* The Hogarth Press, London.

Index